Dental Auxiliary's

Encyclopedic Dictionary

Henry E. Karlin, D.D.S.
Muriel K. Trachman, M.A.

Prentice-Hall, Inc.
Englewood Cliffs, New Jersey

Prentice-Hall International, Inc., *London*
Prentice-Hall of Australia, Pty. Ltd., *Sydney*
Prentice-Hall Canada, Inc., *Toronto*
Prentice-Hall of India Private Ltd., *New Delhi*
Prentice-Hall of Japan, Inc., *Tokyo*
Prentice-Hall of Southeast Asia Pte. Ltd., *Singapore*
Whitehall Books, Ltd., Wellington, *New Zealand*
Editora Prentice-Hall do Brasil Ltda., *Rio de Janeiro*
Prentice-Hall Hispanoamericana, S.A., *Mexico*

This book is a reference work based on
research by the author. The opinions
expressed herein are not necessarily those of
or endorsed by the publisher. The directions
stated in this book are in no way to be
considered as a substitute for consultation
with a duly licensed doctor.

Library of Congress Cataloging-in-Publication Data
Karlin, Henry E. (Henry Edward)
    Dental auxiliary's encyclopedic dictionary.

    1. Dentistry—Practice—Dictionaries.   2. Dentistry—
Dictionaries.   3. Dental auxiliary
personnel—Diction-
aries.   I. Trachman, Muriel K. (Muriel Karlin)
II. Title.   [DNLM: 1. Dental
Auxiliaries—encyclopedias.
2. Dentistry—encyclopedias.   WU 13 k18d]
RK60.5.K36   1986   617.6'003'21   85-16992

ISBN 0-13-198565-5

Printed in the United States of America

Dedication

We dedicate this book,
with our love,
to Debbie and Alexis Nicole Karlin,
Lisa Karlin
and Emmanuel Trachman

A Practical Guide for the Office Manager, Dental Assistant and Hygienist

Dental Auxiliary's Encyclopedic Dictionary is the volume every dental office should have. It is valuable to the office manager, to the dental assistant, and to the dental hygienist. This book contains two sections: The first consists of procedures which auxiliaries must know to function efficiently; the second is a glossary of definitions of words and terms to which every staff member will refer.

The purpose of the *Dental Auxiliary's Encyclopedic Dictionary* is to help the staff function more effectively and competently, always remembering that their time, as that of the dentist, is valuable. Teaching each dental staff member how to make patients feel comfortable and important will help build the dental practice and constantly increase its potential.

This book may be used to train new personnel and to upgrade the skills of experienced dental employees. For example, the office manager can learn billing procedures that will make the collection of fees easier. The dental assistant can become more proficient in the recognition of instruments, thereby increasing the productivity of the dentist. The hygienist will become better equipped to teach home care by studying the entries in this book.

Another feature of Section I is the series of first aid procedures which the staff may need to know in the event of an emergency.

Still another area covered is practice building—with a variety of techniques that may be used to increase patient volume. All of these procedures have been tested and proven in the practice environment.

iv

Furthermore, the staff will find in these pages instructions and assistance in filling out the scores of forms that are constantly being done in dental offices throughout the nation.

One more feature is the forms which may be used "as is," or changed to suit the needs of the office. These include an inventory-control form, an employment-application form, a fee-computation form, a patient health-history form, a daily record of production and collection, a recall form, a series of letters for various situations, and others.

Section II provides all of the terms necessary for use in keeping records and filling out forms. Since nearly every patient has an insurance plan, this has become a very important task in a busy office, and one which can be speeded up by having this ready reference.

Such terms as the following are included:

amalgam—an alloy restoration prepared by mixing silver alloy and mercury

apicoectomy—the surgical removal of the root and abscess of a diseased tooth. This requires going through tissue and bone

dentin—the softer and more sensitive portion of the tooth lying beneath the enamel

extrusion—a super eruption of a tooth when the opposing tooth is lost

inlay—a cast gold restoration known for strength and durability

mandibular—referring to the lower jaw

The *Dental Auxiliary's Encyclopedic Dictionary* may be relied upon for easy reference and valuable information. Its use will save time and earn big dividends, as well as provide information the dentist might be called upon to give to his auxiliary personnel. This volume will, we are sure, prove to be one of the most useful for the dental office manager, the assistant, and the hygienist.

Acknowledgments

Many individuals helped with the preparation of this book, and they are too numerous to mention. However, we would be remiss if we did not express our thanks to the following:

We gratefully appreciate the contributions made by these dentists for reviewing the manuscript while it was in preparation:

Dr. Eugene Atlas, Staten Island, N.Y.

Dr. Harry I. Carter, St. Thomas, U.S.V.I.

Dr. Kenneth C. Fordham, II., Lionville, Pa.

Dr. George Reskakis, Forest Hills, N.Y.

Dr. Marvin J. Robinson, St. Thomas, U.S.V.I.

Dr. Harry G. Sacks, St. Louis, Missouri

Dr. Stanley Weiss, Cedarhurst, N.Y.

The staff of the East End Family Health Center, St. Thomas, U.S.V.I. and especially:

Ms. M. Bonelli, R.D.H.,

Ms. Patricia Connor

Ms. Valencia James

Dental assistants Ms. Judy Perlman, Cedarhurst, N.Y., Ms. Marguerite Roussine, Cedarhurst, N.Y.

To Ms. C. White, of Staten Island, N.Y.: our thanks for her painstaking work in doing the final revision of the manuscript.

Contents

Contents

Contents

Contents

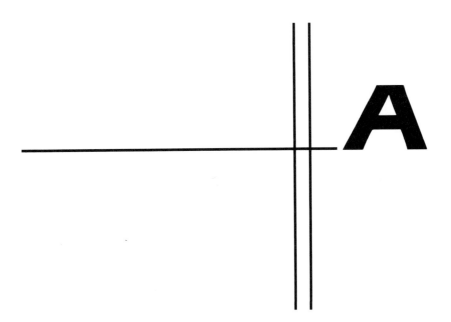

Absence of staff.   Absence of staff members may cause hardship for the others. There are ways in which this hardship may be lessened, but not eliminated.

Do not stay out unless you are absolutely unable to work. Some doctors give bonuses based on perfect attendance, and you may want to discuss this with your employer. Of course you are not expected to go to work when you are ill, but other absences should be avoided if at all possible.

Each staff member should be able to fill in for the others. This requires everyone learning enough of the other's work to be able to handle the essential portions, if and when it becomes necessary. Familiarity with the procedure manual can be a great help in this case.

The dental office manager should be able to assist the doctor if the assistant is absent, and the assistant should be able to make appointments and receive patients in the absence of the office manager.

Another means of avoiding undue hardships is to have part-time employees who are capable of filling in when the full-time staff members are absent. Such "part-timers" can do maintenance or seasonal work such as sending Christmas cards, even though each employee is present.

In the event that you must be out, make arrangements with other staff members to perform your essential duties, so that the office runs as smoothly as possible. If you can take care of your affairs in several hours, ask for the necessary time rather than taking the full day off to do them.

A smoothly running office makes your job that much easier!

ADA. The American Dental Association is a national organization founded in 1840 to improve the health of the public and to promote the art and science of dentistry. Today it has over 116,000 members, with headquarters in Chicago.

The ADA carries on various programs of dental research, inspects and accredits dental schools, and through its committees, accredits auxiliary personnel and hospital dental departments. It reviews legislative and executive proposals affecting dentistry, and produces materials for dental-health education.

The Association publishes the *Journal of the ADA* monthly. Write the American Dental Association, 212 East Chicago Avenue, Chicago, IL. 60611.

ADAA. The American Dental Assistants Association was founded in 1924. It had its origins in Nebraska, where a state association existed from 1917. In 1921 Juliette Southard organized the New York society, and in 1923 she and Jessie Ellsworth, president of the Chicago and Cook County Dental Assistants Association requested aid from members of the **American Dental Association.** They received permission to register all women attending the ADA convention in Cleveland. Fifteen enthusiastic dental assistants were present and elected a committee that laid the groundwork for the formation of a new national association the next year at the ADA convention in Dallas. Juliette Southard was "chairman" and Jessie Ellsworth "vice-chairman" of the committee that worked closely with the then president of the ADA, Dr. John P. Buckley, and others.

When the **ADAA** was incorporated on March 17, 1925 in Illinois, it had four state associations, seven local societies, and about 200 members. Today it has more than 20,000 members consisting of chairside assistants, receptionists, office managers and dental-assisting educators. The organization now has headquarters in Chicago, plus a full-time staff.

The **ADAA** offers to its members the following services: professional liability insurance, accidental death and dismemberment insurance, two free continuing-education courses a year (which enable the dental assistant to renew national certification and state registration, in most states), legal information regarding job-related legal questions and group insurance coverage. There is a member loan program enabling one to borrow up to $5,000 on one's signature. Members receive *The Dental Assistant*, a magazine containing educational articles, practical suggestions, tips and special features, and *Focus*, the national newsletter that provides timely information about pending legislation and Association Activities. There are also state and local newsletters.

One very important aspect of the work of the ADAA is its legislation representation on the state and federal levels. It helps state dental assistant associations by drafting bills and writing and delivering testimony before state boards of dentistry and state legislatures. In Washington it works on the passage of such bills as the Consumer-Patient Radiation Health and Safety Act.

The **ADAA** is the professional organization of dental assistants that has worked for over 60 years to help the dental assistant to develop from an untrained and unskilled office worker into a well-educated auxiliary, knowledgeable about scientific and technical principles, cognizant of the dentist's needs in operatory procedures, and capable of performing many intraoral functions herself.

The **ADAA** has headquarters at 666 North Lake Shore Drive, Chicago, IL 60611.

Advertisements received. You should set the office policy with your employer in regard to the actions he or she wishes you to take; never ignore his or her wishes.

Review all ads carefully. Generally, you can determine which ads to keep and show to your employer, and which to discard.

Allergy

All samples of products are to be given to the doctor, unless you are requested to do otherwise. He or she may wish to distribute certain ones to patients, but this should be done only after you are instructed to do so.

Allergy.   An allergy is a reaction to certain materials in the environment that do not cause the same reaction in others. The materials are called allergens or antigens; they may be any of the following:

> materials inhaled, such as pollen, fungi, dust, smoke, cosmetics, perfumes, and other strong odors
>
> medicines taken internally, such as antibiotics
>
> foods, such as wheat, milk, eggs, fish, nuts, chocolate, strawberries, and pork
>
> infectious materials, such as bacteria, fungi, parasites, and viruses
>
> skin and mucous membrane contactants, such as plants, animals, jewelry, cosmetics, furs, and leather
>
> atmospheric conditions, such as heat, cold, sunlight, and pressure

These antigens may cause two types of reactions. One is the skin breaking out in rashes or hives. The other is respiratory—sneezing, wheezing, and difficulty in breathing.

Patients should be questioned as follows: "Do any of the following apply to you?"

1. Does any medicine applied externally, especially those containing anesthetics, antibiotics, and so on, cause an allergic reaction?
2. List months or seasons when allergic attacks occur.
3. Specify type of reaction—skin or respiratory.
4. Discuss onset of the attack—slow or quick.
5. Mention frequency of attack.
6. Discuss possible allergens.
7. List means by which relief is obtained.
8. State whether attack occurs at the same time as emotional upset.

9. Specify the environment in which most time is spent.
10. Discuss the effect of the following on the patient:
    a. fatigue
    b. excitement
    c. anxiety
    d. overeating
    e. chilling
11. List other illnesses.

This information should be brought to the attention of your doctor.

Ammonia, aromatic.   In the event of a patient fainting, or feeling faint, no dental office should be without capsules that, when snapped, give a whiff of ammonia. *Vaporale*, marketed by the *Burroughs Wellcome Company*, Research Triangle Park, NC 27709, is such a product. It offers fast, effective first aid, and is very convenient to keep on hand.

Anesthesia.   It is the job of the dental assistant to prepare, deliver to the dentist, and dispose of anesthetics used in dental procedures.

There are a variety of drugs the dentist may choose from. The most common one is lidocaine hydrochloride (known to the public as "novacaine"), which contains, in addition to the anesthetic itself, a minute amount of epinephrine, which constricts the blood vessels. Some patients cannot tolerate this substance, and will require a "nonvasoconstricting" anesthetic. One anesthetic without epinephrine is carbocaine.

Your employer will alert you to what is stocked in the office, and when it is needed.

Dental anesthetics are packaged in glass tubes called "carpules" that have a rubber stopper at one end and a metal collar with a plastic center at the other.

Dental syringes usually do not have an attached needle, but have a threaded hub at the end opposite the plunger where a disposable needle may be screwed in.

To load and prepare the syringe, first remove the plastic cap that covers the threaded part of the disposable needle and screw it into the hub of the syringe. Leave the longer cover of the needle in place and check to make sure that the end projecting into the syringe is still straight. Then, retract (pull back) the plunger of the syringe and slip the carpule of anesthesia into the syringe. The end of the carpule with the rubber stopper belongs at the opposite end of the syringe from the needle, and the plastic diaphragm of the capsule should be punctured by the end of the needle that is projecting into the syringe. Recheck to make sure that the carpule has been punctured and the needle remains straight inside it.

If the syringe is an aspirating type, there will be a metal barb at the end of the plunger that must be hooked into the rubber stopper. To do this, gently tap the plunger so the hook engages the rubber stopper.

The disposable needle should be re-covered before being thrown out to prevent accidents.

Be aware that carpules occasionally shatter when being removed from a syringe. It is good practice to avoid holding the syringe in front of your face when emptying it, to minimize the risk of eye injury.

Some dentists use a preinjection topical agent to numb the tissue before giving the shot. You may be expected to dispense the topical anesthetic to the dentist. If so, simply insert the end of a cotton swab into the topical gel and hand it to your employer.

Anesthesia, patient reaction to. It is possible your doctor may leave the room after a patient has been given anesthesia. The patient may react adversely. It is one of the assistant's functions to remain in the operatory and observe the patient. Symptons which may be observed are:

fainting
difficulty opening the jaw
swelling with blood
swelling with a watery fluid
tingling sensation
heavy breathing

If you observe any one or more of these symptoms, or the patient tells you he or she is having them, inform the doctor immediately.

After having been given anesthesia, patients should be permitted to rinse their mouths because anesthesia often has a bad taste.

Announcements. Announcements are an acceptable way of keeping the doctor's name in public. They may be sent under conditions such as:

entering practice
opening a second office
entering a partnership or group practice
change of address
change of hours
entering or returning from the armed forces
assuming another doctor's practice
entering a specialty

All cards, regardless of the main message, should carry the doctor's name, address, telephone number, office hours, and field of specialization if there is one.

Announcements may be mailed to anyone the doctor designates. Generally they are not mailed to people the doctor does not know, but this is not a rule. Since the announcement serves as a type of advertisement, it certainly may be used for this purpose. It may also be sent to other doctors, hospitals, and business organizations.

Answering service. The doctor's answering service is very important to the smooth functioning of the office.

Instructions should be given to the service by the doctor in regard to how they must respond to patient's inquiries, how they handle emergencies, and if they are to make appointments.

Each morning of a working day, either the office manager or the assistant should telephone the answering service to get all of the messages which have been taken. These should be recorded in a daily log book so that they are available permanently; this avoids the loss of messages which can occur when they are written on slips of paper.

Some of the messages require immediate telephone replies to the caller. Others may need a specific response from the doctor, and will be responded to as soon as he or she can be consulted.

Before closing the office for the day, the answering service must be notified so that the operator will take all incoming calls. The same notification is necessary when the office is closed for lunch.

Answering service log book. These are the headings that should appear in your book:

Date	Caller & Phone Number	Nature of Call	Action Taken

It is advisable to use a large ledger for this purpose, so that each entry can be written in easily and completely.

A standard-sized notebook can be used for the purpose, but use a double page, so that plenty of space is available to you.

This type of recording can be very valuable when you have to backtrack for information.

Antibiotics. An antibiotic is a substance produced by living microorganisms that is capable of inhibiting the growth of, or destroying, bacteria and other microorganisms. Antibiotics that inhibit growth of microorganisms are termed bacteriostatic: Erythromycin and tetracycline are two examples of bacteriostatic antibiotics. Penicillin, which destroys microorganisms, is an example of bacteriocidal antibiotics.

When administering or prescribing any antibiotic, it is vital to consult the medical history and question the patient about any reaction he or she may have had to an antibiotic in the past. An allergic reaction may manifest itself as: Breaking out in hives or a rash, swelling of the extremities, convulsions, or in extreme cases, anaphylactic shock. In general, oral administration (as a tablet, capsule or liquid) of an antibiotic is least likely to generate a severe reaction, as the drug is absorbed into the bloodstream most slowly this way. Patients who have experienced an allergic reaction to a given antibiotic usually remember this, and so will be able to tell you this when asked. However, even if the previous response to a drug was negative, it is always possible that the patient may become allergic, and patients should be cautioned accordingly.

The most commonly prescribed antibiotic is the oral form of penicillin—Penicillin VK. It may be administered for a variety of situations: for patients with a medical history of rheumatic heart disease, congenital heart disease or any type of heart prosthesis such as artificial valves; diabetic patients who present dental or periodontal abscesses, or after extractions to prevent subsequent infection. Patients who are allergic to penicillin are usually given erythromycin.

Antibiotics sometimes have side effects, and may cause diarrhea or nausea in some people. For this reason, it is important that when they are administered to patients, full instructions accompany the prescription. These instructions should be gone over verbally as well as in writing

Anxiety—alleviating patient's. Patient anxiety is something you must deal with almost constantly. Patients frequently come into the office in pain. It is necessary that you be as supportive as possible. You can do this in a number of ways:

1. Explain to the patient in pain that the doctor will see him or her as soon as possible. Inform the doctor that the patient has arrived.

2. Explain all procedures that the patient will undergo so he or she knows what to expect, and so that there will be no surprises. Your employer may wish to have some printed material on hand to give to patients, and you can use this as the basis for your personal explanation.

3. If you see a person who is very anxious, a gentle touch on the arm or shoulder may be helpful; hand holding and eye contact can also be reassuring.

4. When a patient must wait for the doctor longer than five minutes in the operatory, supply a magazine or newspaper. It is important that the patient's mind be occupied.

9

5. If the patient is kept waiting, walk into the room frequently to say a few words or, if you can devote the time, engage him or her in conversation.

6. Inform the doctor if any particular patient is abnormally anxious; he or she can then act accordingly.

7. If a procedure which is unpleasant must be performed, tell the patient about it so that he or she knows what to expect. The fewer surprises the anxious patient receives, the better. However, do not ever use words such as "hurt," "pain," "painful," "pull a tooth" or any others that will increase the patient's anxiety.

8. If a patient is very anxious, inform the chair-side assistant, asking her to reassure the patient during treatment. When appropriate, the assistant should say, "The doctor is almost finished now. Try to relax."

9. Encourage anxious patients to breathe deeply; tell them it will help them to relax. Not all will find this helpful, but some of them will.

10. If a patient seems to want to cry, don't try to stop him or her. Words such as "If you feel like crying, go right ahead," can often help, and the tears serve as a release for some of the tension.

11. Some emergency patients may benefit from being anesthetized immediately (if this is possible) or being given a pain-killer or tranquilizer. Before doing this, discuss office policy with your doctor.

12. It is not a good idea to sit an emergency or anxious patient in a vacant operatory unless an assistant or yourself can keep them company.

Remember that anxiety may stem from previous bad experiences and can be a major factor in the patient's overall perception of your health care. Solicitous and perceptive handling of these patients can be an excellent way of gaining new patients and referrals.

Appointment book. Specific needs dictate the use of an appointment book that will make the scheduling of patients as efficient as possible. When purchasing your book, look for these characteristics:

1. A looseleaf binder allows you to flip pages back and forth easily and can contain any given number of months. These pages should be tabbed, so that you can find what you are looking for easily.
2. The book should lie flat.
3. Each space should allot 15 minutes of time.
4. You should be able to see one week at a time without flipping pages.
5. Each patient entry should include the name, phone number, service to be given, and time allotted for it.

One person should be responsible for keeping the book, although other personnel may consult it as well.

By writing in the book in pencil, changes can be made simply by erasing, rather than crossing out.

The doctor should mark into the appointment book several months in advance (or as long ahead as is possible) when the office will be closed. He or she should also indicate the times set aside for lunch, and for the treatment of emergencies, and these should be so marked.

The policy for the scheduling of the most challenging types of work, which require the most effort, should be established so that the assistant can schedule those patients when the doctor wishes to treat them. This eliminates undue strain on the doctor and the entire staff.

Develop a type of shorthand for notations in the book. This will enable you to save both time and space. Tape a copy of the symbols used in the front of the book so that in the event you are not available, the notations can be understood by others.

Appointment breaking, working with. The patient who breaks appointments is the cause of lost revenue as well as aggravation. This type of person can prove to be a real nuisance, and must be dealt with.

It is possible that people who do this are simply thoughtless. In conversation, they should be told, "We have an office policy that requires us to charge for all broken appointments. I've checked with the doctor, and this time we will not charge you, but next time we must." Continue this conversation by telling the patient, "It is very important that you keep your appointment because your dental condition deteriorates. You're here because you want your mouth to be as attractive and healthy as possible. By not having your work done on schedule, you are seriously interfering with your treatment."

It is also entirely possible that patients are very frightened. Talk with them, and try to determine if this is the case. If it is, suggest premedication. Tell them there are many patients who felt this way. The doctor gave them something that helped them, and they were able to finish their work as planned. The medication, you can explain to them, is mild and non-habit-forming.

Appointment cards. Appointment cards are usually the standard business-card size, 3½ inches by 2 inches. Write one card for each patient, and give it to him or her. They should contain the following information:

> the doctor's name
>
> address
>
> telephone number
>
> two blank spaces

Use the first blank space for the patient's name, and the second for the date and time of the next appointment. If an appointment is made on the telephone, mail an appointment card to serve as a reminder.

Some dentists prefer to use colored stock, rather than a white card; this is, of course, a matter of personal preference.

Some dentists include a statement about cancellations on the card, indicating whether or not a charge will be made for broken appointments.

Appointments. The efficient scheduling of patients is crucial to the efficient management of a busy dental office.

Guidelines must be established by the dentist in regard to the amount of time to be allotted to each patient. For example, a full examination requires more time than a follow-up visit.

12

An appointment book should be selected that fulfulls the needs of your office. It may have time-allocation spaces for full hours, half hours, or quarter hours.

One person should be in charge of the appointment book, and have responsibility for it.

Indicate appointments in pencil, so that they may be changed easily.

In making appointments, fill in the following information:

1. Patient's name
2. Telephone number
3. Problem or nature of the visit
4. If the patient is new, the name of the person who made the referral.

Make the appointments only during regular office hours unless you are instructed to by your employer to do otherwise.

Whenever the doctor will be away from the office during his regular hours, block the time out so that it is impossible for you to schedule patients during that time.

With the doctor's permission, leave one schedule slot open in the morning, and one in the afternoon. Leaving slots open enables you to give emergency appointments when necessary. One appointment slot should also be left open for returning phone calls at the end of the day.

Assignment of insurance payments by the patient to the doctor. When patients assign payment by their insurance company to the doctor, you should make sure they understand exactly what has been done. Normally the payment will be sent to your doctor for the amount of money the insurance covers. The doctor will then bill the patient for the remainder of the fee.

Should the assigned payment not be paid directly or fully by the insurance company, explain to the patient that he or she will be billed. In fact, he or she should be billed until the payment assigned has been paid by the insurance company.

Explain all of this in advance. If you fail to do so, certain patients may become upset because they think (and say) "My bill was paid by the insurance company." Make sure they understand whether the entire bill would be covered, or only a portion of it.

It is to your advantage to have the insurance payment sent directly to your office, rather than to the patient, who will then have to send it to you. Many times patients hold up these payments to you, in spite of the fact that the checks are made out to the doctor.

Asthma. Asthma is considered to be a harmful and disabling respiratory disease. Patients who suffer from asthma may have attacks at any time, caused by a closing down of the small bronchial tubes in the lungs. This causes a wheezing or whistling sound when the patient breathes.The most common type of asthma is caused by allergic reactions, generally to ordinary household substances such as dust, pollens, or certain foods.

Asthma attacks are often associated with periods of heavy emotional strain or physical exertion.

If a patient informs you he or she has asthma, call this to your doctor's attention.

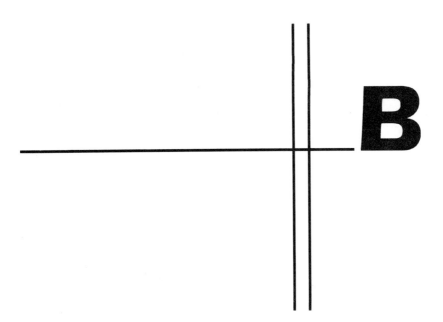

Bankruptcy, patients declaring.   As economic times change, it is possible for more and more patients to go into bankruptcy. Money owed to a dentist is in the same category as any other debts.

There are two types of bankruptcy. In either event the relevant laws are federal, and a person who files for bankruptcy becomes a ward of the state. When a person files a straight petition of bankruptcy, no creditor can attempt to collect money owed to him. The creditors are listed on a form which may be obtained from the referee involved in the case.

In a wage-earner's bankruptcy, the person pays a fixed amount to the trustee in bankruptcy, who, in turn, pays it to the creditors. This action is all that can be done. Once bankruptcy has been filed, the person's salary cannot be attached or garnished.

When either type of bankruptcy has been filed for, the doctor is usually one of the last persons to be paid. Fortunately, to date, personal bankruptcies of this type are relatively unusual. It is far more frequent to find patients who are slow payers, or who pay the doctor last. In that case collection procedures are appropriate.

Bases—liners and temporaries. After cutting a tooth, the dentist may feel the need to medicate it before filling it. This may be to insulate the dentin, form new dentin, or add bulk to the dentin for a more retentive filling or crown. The assistant should be familiar with the uses of, indications for, and methods of mixing and dispensing the necessary materials.

Calcium hydroxide (dycal) is probably the most frequently used base. It promotes growth of dentin, and is used as a pulp-capping material in near exposures or small pulp exposures. It is packaged in two small tubes. Equal amounts of base and accelerator are squeezed onto a small paper pad, and mixed with a special instrument, which is then wiped off and handed to the dentist along with a pad. The doctor dips the tip of the instrument in the material and places it in the prepared tooth. This must be done speedily as the material sets quickly.

Another frequently used base is cement, of which a number of types are available. If the cavity has destroyed a lot of tooth structure, cement is used to provide insulation between the remaining tooth and the filling; it is also used for cementing crowns, bridges and inlays. Zinc-phosphate cement (ZOP) is dispensed as a liquid and a powder. It is mixed on a glass slab (preferably chilled) with a cement spatula. The liquid part of the cement is phosphoric acid, which may inflame a pulp, so, when mixing, as much powder as possible should be incorporated in the liquid to minimize the acidity of the cement. Mixing over as wide an area as possible of the slab should be employed to prevent excess acidity. The cement is ready for use when the mass of the mixture forms a string when lifted by the spatula. For crowns and bridges, six drops of liquid are used per abutment or crown; for a base under a filling, the proper amount should be estimated.

Various nonacid cements such as carboxylate cement are also commercially available. Carboxylate cement, known under the proprietary name of *Durelon*, is also a liquid-powder system, and is dispensed with a special scoop that comes with the kit and an eyedropper. It is mixed on the glass slab to a creamy consistency and, like ZOP, transferred to the mouth on a dental instrument that resembles an amalgam plugger.

Cavity liners are substances placed on the tooth to seal the cut dentin. These are liquids, and are often called "varnishes."

The most common liner in use is called *Copalite,* and is a gum resin. It comes in a bottle and is carried to the tooth by a cotton pellet held in a pair of college pliers (tweezers) that are first dipped in the bottle.

Temporary fillings are placed for a variety of reasons, including medication of a sensitive tooth, during pulp therapy where the tooth must be opened repeatedly, and while waiting for laboratory work such as inlays or crowns. For sedation of painful teeth, the filling material of choice is a zinc oxide-eugenol mixture. This mixture is available commercially in kit form or the ingredients may be purchased in bulk from a drug or supply store. Eugenol (oil of cloves), imparts its characteristic smell to the dental office. Both forms of this temporary filling are mixed on a glass slab to a thick but pliable consistency. Cotton fibers may be incorporated into the ZOE to increase its strength. ZOE is commonly mixed before any patients are seen and kept in a humidifier until needed.

If a tooth must be reopened, such as during endodontic therapy, a solid filling material that is easy to remove is often the filling of choice. One common material in use is Cavit G., which is packaged in a glass jar and dispensed on the end of a plastic instrument. Cavit is another filling material, and is packaged in a tube. Cavit is a temporary filling of choice when the dental nerve is still present; Cavit G when the nerve has been removed.

If an anterior tooth is to be temporized, acrylic is mixed in a dappen dish. The powder is placed in the dish, and an eyedropper is used to saturate the powder with a liquid, which is then mixed with a spatula. The mixture should be creamy and firm.

Billing—confidentiality. The financial matters between your office and every patient are highly confidential. Be sure they are kept that way, since it is possible you could be involved in a slander suit if confidentiality is not observed.

Never discuss one patient's financial affairs with anyone else, for any reason whatsoever.

Never discuss financial matters concerning one patient within hearing of another. (If your office is within hearing

Billing information

range of the waiting room, suggest to your employer that some means of achieving privacy be installed.)

Never allow a person who is employed in your office to do work that may give them access to patient's financial records or outstanding bills. This rule includes part-timers, and may even pertain to other members of the staff.

Billing information. Use the form that follows; it should be included in the patient's folder. It is very important to include this in his or her record.

BILLING INFORMATION

Patient's Name _____

Address _____

Telephone Number _____

Social Security Number _____

Employer _____

Insurance Coverage

    Company _____

    Insurance Connected with Employer _____

    Other Policies _____

_____

_____

Person To Whom Bills Are to Be Sent _____

_____

Address _____

Relationship to Patient _____

Billing systems; commercial. The *Accounts Receivable Management System* from **Control-o-fax** is a system that is simple to use, but which expands to meet your needs. "Pegboard forms" give you a daily record of every patient transaction from the

18

time the patients walk in the door, receive treatment and leave. The "Superbill" lets one person process an insurance copy, a receipt and an appointment slip all in one writing. It encourages patients to pay as they leave, and third-party insurance claims get paid faster because they're processed at the time of treatment.

The billing part of the service handles monthly billing. You complete the basic paperwork, and your unpaid ledger cards are microfilmed, your current statements are mailed and all past-due accounts are specially flagged for your attention.

For information contact **Control-o-fax,** Box 778, Waterloo, IA 50704.

For new dentists, the *Practice Builder* is available. It contains all the printed forms needed to get the system started at a reasonable cost.

Blind patients, behavior toward. Blind patients require special attention, both from you and the doctor; if you can schedule them on a relatively light day, it is well worth doing so.

Of course you would allow a person who has a seeing eye dog to bring the animal into the office. There are some persons who, while legally blind, have some sight. If you can determine how much, you will know how much assistance to offer. If not, then here are some suggestions:

As the person enters your waiting room, get up and go over to him. Shake hands and say "How do you do, Mr. Jones. Dr. Brown will see you very soon. I'm his office manager Ms. Smith. Please sit down here."

Another person may accompany the blind patient. If so, be sure you speak directly to the patient. Speaking to the other person makes the blind person feel inadequate.

When the patient goes into the operatory, tell him in a soft voice exactly what to do. For example, "The examining room is fifteen steps straight down the hall. Then we must turn to the left into the room." Walk very slowly just a step ahead of him.

Keep watch, and if the patient must be guided, take his arm gently and steer him. Do not do this unless it is necessary or if you are going up or down stairs. If the patient uses a cane, he may not require this type of assistance. Introduce him to the dental assistant.

After entering the room, bring the patient to the chair and put his hands on it, both on the seat and the back. In this way he is able to orient himself to it.

Before you leave to return to your desk, tell the person, "The doctor will be with you as soon as possible. Is there anything further I can do for you?" Wait for an answer. If it is negative, excuse yourself by saying, "Please excuse me, I have to get back to my desk." This lets the patient know he will be alone in the room until the doctor enters.

After the doctor has examined or treated the patient, the dental assistant should guide him back to the waiting room, and review the instructions the doctor has given him.

Offer your assistance by asking "Is there anything else we can do for you?" For example, the patient may want you to make a telephone call, or request a taxi.

Say "goodbye" in a friendly manner and escort the patient to the door.

Busy days, preparation for. Every dental office has peak times—when you are extremely busy, with a full compliment of patients, a constantly ringing telephone, and an emergency now and then. What can you do to make these times easier?

1. Do as much work in nonpeak times as you possible can. Sit down and figure out what time-consuming jobs you have to do—and when you can best do them. If you have part-timers, assign some of this work to them.

2. Prepare your own forms to cover as many situations as possible.

3. Have forms that patients must fill out ready for them. When carbon copies are necessary, prepare those "packages" beforehand.

4. Pull records for those patients the doctor will see as soon as you start work for the day. Refile them either at the end of the day or the next morning.

5. Use an appointment book that is large enough for you to write in, and read back, easily. One-quarter inch spaces are far too small, and make your work more difficult.

6. Have a list of frequently called telephone numbers readily available (See entry "Telephone lists, essential").

20

7. Do your filing every day. Never let it pile up—if you do, it can hamper the smooth running of your office.

8. Have all medications clearly labelled and stored in alphabetical order when possible.

9. Never leave a single area of the office dirty or untidy. Each room should be cleaned before closing the office for the night. All waste baskets should be emptied and the garbage taken out.

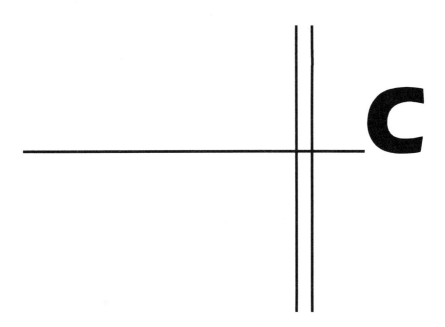

Calling patients from the waiting room. While some dentists prefer to call patients into their offices or examining rooms personally, others prefer to have their assistants do this.

If you have this task, ask the doctor how he prefers you to do this. If you are to say "Mrs. Smith, the doctor is ready to see you now," it should be said with a smile and a friendly nod.

Avoid giving the patient the impression he or she is just a number, and the situation is similar to that of a "bakery waiting line".

If your waiting room is crowded, and your list or schedule shows the next patient to be seen in Jenny Jones, but you have no idea which person Jenny is, look at the charts you have in front of you. Find out Jenny's age, weight and height, and then you may be able to spot her. If not, say the name, "Mrs. Jenny Jones," while looking down at the record until she rises and comes towards you.

While some doctors do call their patients by their first names, unless there is a special reason for you to do so , do not follow this procedure. If the person is someone you are socially friendly with, then, and only then, is this permissible.

Cancellation of appointments by the doctor.   Whenever it is necessary to cancel appointments, do so as soon as you learn of it.

Telephone the patient. If you cannot reach him, either personally or to leave a message, send a Mailgram.

In speaking to the person, use words to the effect "Dr. X. is taking care of an emergency, and has to cancel all his (her) appointments. We're very sorry to inconvenience you. We can see you _____ (and tell the patient the new time).

If the doctor is to be delayed, courtesy dictates you call the patient and advise him or her of this. No patient should be kept waiting any longer than necessary.

Cancellation of appointments by the patient.   When a first appointment is broken by the patient, immediately offer to make another one. However, explain that appointments are responsibilities, and cancellations are an inconvenience.

Determine, with your doctor, the policy to be followed with patients who repeatedly break appointments. Should they be rescheduled immediately or a month in the future? Should they be charged for the broken appointment?

It is also good policy to note cancellations in the permanent record, in the space allotted to that day's procedure. The patient who calls you to cancel an appointment is not the same as a patient who doesn't show up and fails to call in advance. The latter patient should have "dis-appointment" written in the permanent record and the former, "cancellation." As it is in the best interest of everyone to have all office hours used as productively as possible, you can minimize "downtime" (when the dentist is present but not working) by having alternate patients available on call when a patient who chronically misses his visits is scheduled. Your doctor may offer a discount to those patients who are available on short notice. Discuss this with him or her.

Cash basis accounting.   Taxes are a very important aspect of the business of running a dental practice. The majority of dentists use cash basis accounting, which is based on the concept that only money which is actually received or paid out is considered for accounting purposes for the year of transaction.

Let us say Mrs. Smith sees Dr. X on December 23, 1984. She is billed for $150.00. She does not pay her bill until January 8, 1985. This $150.00 is not part of Dr. X's income for 1984, but is for 1985.

By the same token, if Dr. Y receives an order of office stationery costing $120.00 on December 5, 1984, but pays for it in January 1985, it is part of his or her operating expenses for 1985, not 1984.

Unpaid charges and bills are both important, but are not considered for accounting purposes under this system until they are paid for.

Cash receipts book. This book is used to record all cash received by the dentist from sources other than his patients. For example, these sources might include scrap gold, income from investments or bank dividends. The total of this figure plus that of payments from his patients shows the doctor's income on any particular day.

It is important that a book of this kind be kept, in order to keep the financial records clear. When income from patients is listed in the same book as that from other investments and sources, problems can arise.

Catalogs. It is a very good idea to keep catalogs of dental supplies and equipment in your files so that you may order an item quickly if it is needed.

Examples of companies offering extensive catalogs are

Henry Schein, Inc., 5 Harbor Park Drive, Port Washington, NY 11050

Interstate Drug Exchange, Engineers Hill, Plainview, NY 11803.

Silvermans's, 5 Apollo Rd., Box 368, Plymouth Meeting, PA 19462

Great Lakes, 1550 Herfel Ave., Buffalo, NY 14216.

Centigrade—Fahrenheit equivalents. It may be necessary for you to convert Centigrade temperature readings to Fahrenheit. Remember that $-40°$ Centigrade $= -40°$ Fahrenheit. Water freezes at $0°$ C. and $32°$ F. Water boils at $100°$ C. and $212°$ F.

Certification for dental assistants

To convert degrees F to degrees C, subtract 32 and multiply by $\frac{5}{9}$. For example, to change 212° F to C: $212 - 32 = 180 \times \frac{5}{9} = 100°$ C

To convert degrees C to degrees F, multiply by $\frac{9}{5}$ and add 32. For example, to change 100° C to F: $100 \times \frac{9}{5} = 180 + 32 = 212°$ F.

Centigrade-Fahrenheit Equivalents

Centigrade°	Fahrenheit°
0	32
5	41
10	50
15	59
20	68
25	77
30	86
35	95
37	98.6
39	102.2
40	104
42	107.6
45	113
50	122
55	131
60	140
65	149
70	158
75	167
80	176
85	185
90	194
95	203
100	212

Certification for dental assistants. Becoming a Certified Dental Assistant is one way in which the dental assistant can improve her professional status. She can, for example, use the letters *C.D.A.* (Certified Dental Assistant) after her name. Certification is available through the **Dental Assisting National Board, Inc.,** located at 666 N. Lake Shore Drive, Chicago, IL

60611. There are three areas in which an assistant may be certified: *General Chairside Assisting, Oral and Maxillofacial Surgery Assisting,* and *Dental Practice Management Assisting.*

The requirements to take the examination for certification may be fulfilled in one of several ways. Basically these involve graduation from a dental-assisting program accredited by the **American Dental Association Commission on Dental Accreditation** and having taken a current course in Cardiopulmonary Resuscitation (CPR) with either the **American Heart Association** or the **American Red Cross.** High school graduation plus five years of full-time work experience (10,000 hours) may be substituted for the dental-assisting program. In the case of the certification for *Oral and Maxillosurgery Assisting,* one must have had formal education or more specific work experience.

In addition to fulfilling the requirements specified above, one must take and pass a written examination, consisting of multiple choice and matching questions. Dental charting is required, and the applicants are required to answer test questions based on the completed charting. The questions are oriented to the certification area for which the examination is being taken. All questions pertaining to charting require that the applicant know the Universal tooth numbering system. Applicants will not be allowed to write the conditions to be charted, or to use abbreviations. Test questions require that the applicant be able to differentiate between restorations and carious lesions on the chart.

The examination includes questions on the following topics:

    collection and recording of chairside data

    dental radiology

    chairside dental procedures

    chairside dental materials

    laboratory materials and procedures

    prevention of disease transmission

    patient education and oral health management

    prevention and management of emergencies

    occupational safety

    office management procedures

Examinations are given four times a year—in February, June, October and in August. Test centers are located in every state. Applicants living more than 150 miles from an established testing center may request a special test center to be established closer to the applicant's residence—but such test centers will be opened only during the October testing period. Applicants are notified ten days before the test of the specific date their tests will be given.

The initial certification is earned for a one-year period based on the anniversary date assigned at the time of certification. Certification must be renewed on a periodic basis. Annual recertification is earned through continuing education courses, which are offered in every state, and which must be in a program accredited by the **ADA Commission on Dental Accreditation.** It is also possible to earn multiyear recertification. Unless one is recertified, she is not permitted to use the certifying credential.

For full information, including sample questions of the type to be found on the certifying examination, contact the **Dental Assisting National Board** at the address given at the beginning of this entry.

Chart. The following is a concise dental chart that the author has used in his practice with good results. The upper half of the form provides space for the patient's name, and intra- and extraoral examination results and the oral hygiene classification (that is, presence or absence of calculus deposits and their extent, and space to evaluate the occlusion).

The lower half of the chart is used to transfer the results of the clinical examination. Note that all teeth have space to correspond to the surface where caries or existing restorations are observed. Space for the deciduous dentition is below the symbols for the permanent teeth, and the same location is to be used as the permanent tooth chart for surfaces. In charting the mixed dentition, besides placing an X through an unerupted permanent tooth, a U placed above or below the symbols indicates that the permanent successor is unerupted.

See dental chart on page 29. This is the lower half of the chart.

Sample Dental Chart.

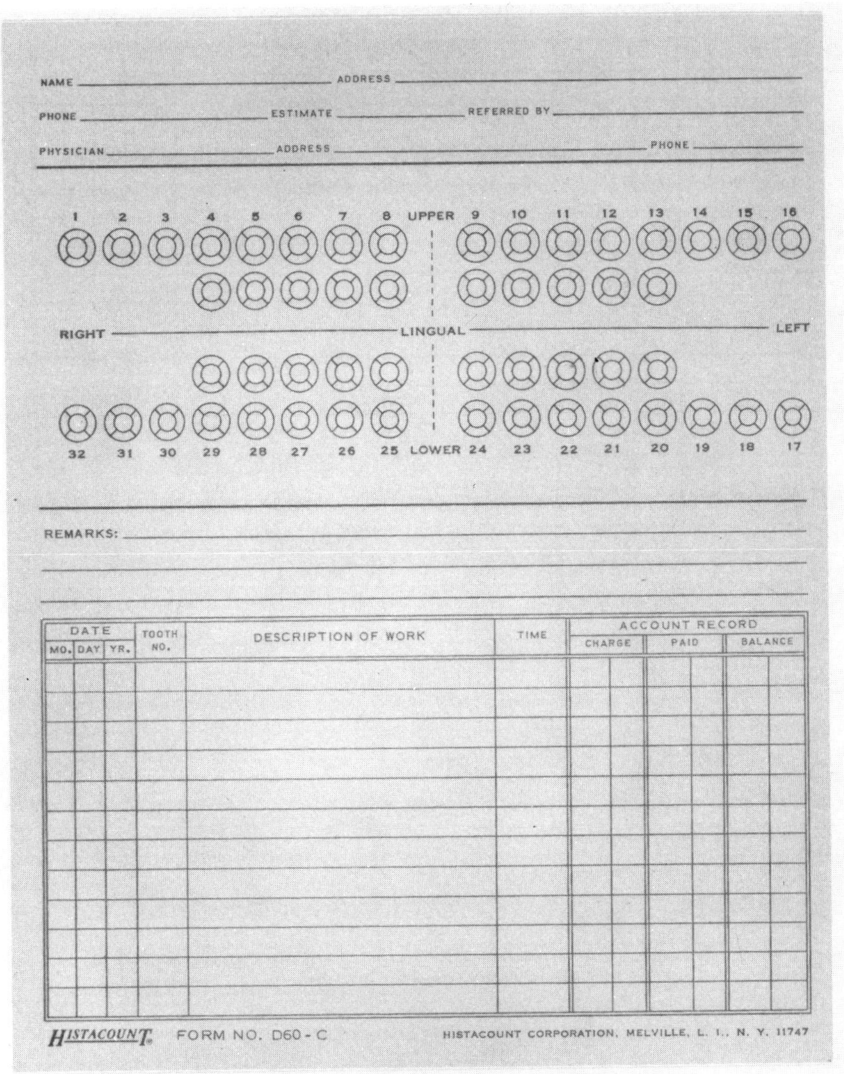

NAME ______ ADDRESS ______

PHONE ______ ESTIMATE ______ REFERRED BY ______

PHYSICIAN ______ ADDRESS ______ PHONE ______

1 2 3 4 5 6 7 8 UPPER 9 10 11 12 13 14 15 16

RIGHT — LINGUAL — LEFT

32 31 30 29 28 27 26 25 LOWER 24 23 22 21 20 19 18 17

REMARKS:

DATE			TOOTH NO.	DESCRIPTION OF WORK	TIME	ACCOUNT RECORD		
MO.	DAY	YR.				CHARGE	PAID	BALANCE

HISTACOUNT FORM NO. D60-C HISTACOUNT CORPORATION, MELVILLE, L. I., N. Y. 11747

Charting. The dental chart is a record of all diagnostic information gathered about a patient's health, recommendations for treatment of any problems encountered, and an ongoing diary of procedures already performed. Charts are legal documents and must be treated with strict confidentiality.

Methods used to file, store and record data on a chart vary from office to office. One of your first responsibilities in any new job is to master the particular format used in the office. Dental assistants should obtain a blank master chart as soon as they are hired and learn as much from it as possible. Remember that you may have to chart from dictation, so first ascertain what numbering system of teeth your office employs. There are

Locations of Teeth for Charting Purposes

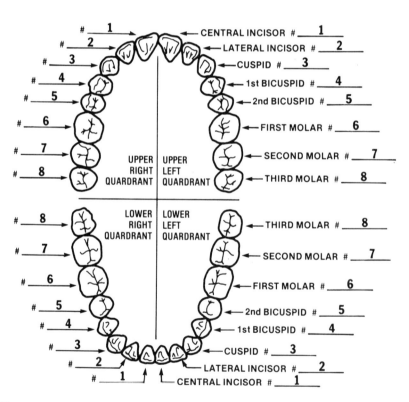

many systems in use today; the system used in the office usually depends on the system your employer learned in dental school.

You should know that all five surfaces of any tooth have a description (Mesial, Distal, Lingual, Buccal (or Facial) and Occlusal (or Incisal)) on the chart. Remember that we all have two sets of teeth, "baby" or primary, and the permanent dentition. There will be space on the chart for representing both.

Most offices also have a conventional shorthand for charting and recording procedures. Often, different color ink is used to represent these findings, and you should make it a priority to master the system and symbols employed. You will soon be able to translate the dental shorthand that your office uses accurately and succinctly.

In general, the more specific a record is of the procedure completed, medications administered or prescribed, and any other pertinant data, the better off your employer is.

Charts, writing up. Be sure that you do all of your charting while the patient is seated in the chair. It is dangerous to try to remember, after a patient has left, what you are supposed to write on his or her chart. Memory is unreliable many times, and it is possible you can omit important information, or even put in the wrong data.

Don't rush while you are charting. This procedure is very important, and errors can make a difference. This is your area of responsibility, and you must take it seriously. Charts are considered to be legal documents by the courts. Mistakes can come back to haunt you, and since you are dealing with very detailed information, you have to give it your full attention while you're doing it.

Checkbook reconciling. There are very few people whose checkbook balance always matches the balance indicated on their bank statement. Here are instructions for reconciling the two.You may be surprised at how relatively simple this procedure may prove to be, if you perform each step carefully:

Checkbook reconciling

1. You must start with the balance in the checkbook having been reconciled with the previous bank statement. You cannot have made errors and expect to correct them if the statement wasn't in agreement with the checkbook to begin with. (In really severe cases it may be necessary to go back to the very beginning of the account—or have an experienced bookkeeper discover the error.)

2. Place all of the checks you received in numerical order.

3. Go through and find each check that is outstanding. Write those numbers on a sheet of paper. (Some bank statements have a place for this.)

4. Go back to your checkbook and next to each number write the amount of the check.

5. Total the amounts of item 3. This is the amount of money still in the bank, although checks have been written for it.

6. Next find the notation on the bank statement for each check that cleared and put a small mark next to it on the bank statement. All of the checks should be listed on the statement. Add these checks.

7. Then check your deposit slips against the notation of deposits. All deposits should have been credited to your account.

8. If you have a deposit slip but have not been credited with that deposit, hold it aside.

9. Check the bank statement to find any charges for service. If there are some, deduct this from the last total in your checkbook.

10. Write down the final balance shown by the bank. Add any deposits you weren't credited for (Item 8).

> Final bank balance
> + Uncredited deposits
> Total — funds in bank
> −Checks not cleared
> Actual bank balance

This bank balance should equal the balance in your checkbook. What if it doesn't? How can you find the error?

a. Go over all of the steps above.

   1. Check your arithmetic carefully.

   2. Did you skip a deposit?

3. Did you skip a check?
4. Did you subtract the service charge from the check-book balance?
5. Did you deduct the correct amount when you wrote each check?
6. Look at each check. On the bottom right of the check is a long number. At the extreme right is the amount the bank deducted for that check. Make sure it is equal to the amount for which the check was written.

Many times the arithmetic is at fault, or the service charges were not deducted.

When you have completed reconciling your bank statement and checkbook, then and only then change the total in the checkbook.

If you cannot locate the error, check the bank. While it is relatively rare, bank personnel do make errors.

Checking accounts. Dentists usually have two or more checking accounts.

A. One is personal—for the payment of all personal and living expenses. These include the doctor's personal investments and transactions.
B. Others are business accounts—for all expenses related to the practice. If the practice is incorporated, these accounts will be for the corporation. The doctor will be paid a salary, as will all the other employees of the corporation, out of this account.

All monies paid by patients—whether they are in the form of checks or cash, should be deposited on a regular schedule. Some employers choose to make daily deposits, others less often. Deposits may be made by the doctor, or the member of the staff designated to do so.

The office manager is responsible for all financial matters including writing checks and keeping the checkbook reconciled.

Use a calender to check the date, making sure it is written correctly. (Be especially careful of this at the beginning of a new month or year.)

Check writing

Be sure of the spelling of the recipient's name. Use "Mrs." only if you are using the husband's first name (Mrs. John Jones" or "Mary Jones" but not "Mrs. Mary Jones"). It is unnecessary to write "Mr.," or "Ms."

When filling in the amount, never change a figure. (If need be, void the check.)

The amount of the check is written twice—once in words and once in numbers. These must, of course, be the same.

When writing figures, be sure the numbers are so close to the dollar sign that it is impossible to place another number between your first number and that dollar sign. The number of cents, or two zeroes, are written above the line in smaller figures, and "100" is written below the line (cents are therefore expressed as fractions of the dollar). If you must send a check for less than one dollar, write the word "Only" before the number of cents. ("Only twenty two cents.")

Your doctor will probably wish to sign all checks unless you are delegated to do so.

Check writing. Write all checks in blue-black (*permanent*) nonwashable ink. Print or type your checks if your handwriting is unclear. (Beware of the pens with erasable ink!)

Fill out the stub and then the check, being sure the numbers of the check and the stub are the same. It may be necessary for you to write in these numbers. If so, do this for the entire book of checks, in advance.

Child abuse. Dental personnel are sometimes in the position of being the first professionals to see injuries inflicted on children by parents, siblings, foster parents or other family members. Often these injuries consist of broken teeth, broken jaws, bruises or contusions of the head or face areas.

Discuss with your employer the policy he or she wishes to follow if such abuse is seen. The matter should be referred to the police with the request that it be kept strictly confidential, and that they be asked to "check it out." Since it is the duty of school officials to make such complaints, the parents may be led to believe it is they who have made the complaint.

The frequency of child abuse is on the rise in this country, and the cooperation of every professional is needed to curb it. On the other hand, realize that the upper front teeth are frequently injured in sporting activities such as playing ball, bicycle riding or just "horsing around." Often, the abused child will not admit that he or she is being mistreated. If you suspect a child of being victimized, discuss it with your employer before taking your suspicions to an outside agency.

Children.   The reaction of a child to your office may influence his feelings toward dentists all his life. It is therefore most important that he be conditioned so that the experience is a positive rather than negative one. There are a number of ways in which this may be done.

1. Smile and act affectionately from the minute the child enters the office. Hugs are perfectly appropriate regardless of the child's age. Who doesn't enjoy a hug, providing, of course, it's sincere? Be lavish with your greeting and call the child by name, but add "dear" or "honey" to it.

2. Explain, as well as you can, what is going to happen when the doctor sees the child. If there's going to be pain, tell the youngster, "This may hurt a little." Then, do not fail to add the words, "It's okay to cry if you have to. Of course you may not have to."

Never, ever, lie to a child. You can do great damage if you do.

3. Establish a reward system. This involves having a supply of trinkets, games, etc. on hand to give to the youngsters. Show these to them and tell them, in advance, with a smile,"We give these presents to the best behaved boys and girls." You may prefer to give the child a trinket before work is begun, and then one afterward. Do not, however, allow any child to leave without one. It may be for "being a great patient," or "being a good patient" or "trying hard to be a good patient." But, in order to make this conditioning work, the words "good patient" should be emphasized.

Your attitude, in this regard, is very important. While it cannot overcome actual pain, it can defeat negative feelings of discomfort.

One enterprising pediatrician gave his patients helium-filled balloons. They proved to be a great success—and a good practice builder because his name was printed on them.

4. If your doctor treats a number of children, have books or magazines available for them to look at. Coloring books and crayons are also good to keep in the waiting room. Small toys can be kept there, although this may prove to be expensive.

If the space is available, a separate play area may be set up, and even decorated for the children.

5. Never leave a child alone in the operatory within reach of any instruments. Children are naturally curious, and when unsupervised, may hurt themselves seriously since there are sharp points and easily breakable objects within their reach. It is possible they may break or damage equipment which is expensive and difficult to repair.

If you must leave the operatory, wait until the doctor returns, or call in one of the other staff members, or as a last resort call in the parent.

Children move very quickly and your absence for even a very short time can permit an accident to occur.

Do not give children dental instruments—even for a moment. If your doctor wants the child to see a mirror, hold it in your hand while the child looks at it.

Children, motivating.   The **American Society of Dentistry for Children** has produced a large variety of excellent motivational materials. These include posters, stickers, health activity and coloring books, birthday cards, balloons and certificates ("Official Dentist's Helper Award") that may also be used as a recall notice. For parents they offer such materials as fliers ("Home dental care for the infant"; "Pit and fissure sealants for your child's teeth").

For teachers, there is the "Teacher's Guide/Flip Chart," which can be used by the dentist when speaking to children in grades from kindergarten to third grade.

For your office there is a rubber stamp, 1½ x 1 inch with smiling faces and the words "Stamp out dental neglect." There are newsletters to which you can add your personalized message, slogan buttons ("Look at me! I'm cavity-free."), and slide/type programs ("Child Abuse Alert").

For full information contact the ASDC, 211 E. Chicago Avenue, Suite 920, Chicago, IL 60611.

Christmas cards. Suggest to your employer that he or she send Christmas cards to all patients. This is a relatively inexpensive form of advertising, fostering good public relations.

Many patients display cards they receive. Care in the selection of an appropriate card should be taken. It is possible to use a calendar card, which has the greetings at the bottom. People use the calendar all year, and, as a result, the doctor's name is kept in front of them for all that time.

Humorous cards are another possibility, and we have received many favorable comments on them.

Cleanliness. A dental office should be spotless at all times— regardless of how busy the staff is. Patients can really be "turned off" at the sight of a soiled towel or a spot on the wall. It is necessary to look at your surroundings from the patients' perspective rather than your own when checking for cleanliness.

Wastebaskets should be covered, rather than left open with their contents visible.

To clean spots from walls, use a product such as *Fantastic, Mr. Clean* a similar product. Remember to clean a larger area than just the spot. Blood spots usually respond to cold water.

Floors should be dust mopped, so that there is no sign of any material on them.

When furniture becomes shabby it looks dirty. It is important that this be avoided. Slipcovers may help in this regard. Rugs or carpeting also can give the appearance of being dirty— even if they actually aren't. In the event that these furnishings require replacement, call this to the attention of your employer.

Even the cleanest office may look dingy if the lighting is inadequate. Make sure there are sufficient lights to have the environment look sparkling. If it does not, it is possible your walls require repainting. White walls will give a crisp appearance, but may be too "hospital-like" for your taste. The cool colors—

light blues and greens—are effective. Be sure these colors have not had gray added to them, or brown. Use them in their pure state for best effect.

Floors, while very attractive if highly waxed, are dangerous, and therefore such polishing should be avoided. However, they must be cared for with a less "high-lustre' dressing.

Ceilings should be dust-mopped on a weekly basis, particularly if your office is not in a new building. Cobwebs form very quickly and, again, convey a feeling of uncleanliness.

If you have a problem with any sort of insects, arrange for a periodic visit from an exterminator. These pests can be kept under control.

All of the tasks mentioned above should be incorporated into your daily routines, so that they are never overlooked.

Collecting fees. This is an important part of your job. If patients can be encouraged to pay for their treatment after each visit, the expense of mailing bills is cut down.

As the patient gets ready to leave, you may say pleasantly, "Mr. Smith, the fee for this visit is $x." Then, pick up your receipt book and pen, and wait. Avoid the appearance of annoyance or pressure. You are structuring the situation, and utilizing the power of suggestion. If the payment is not forthcoming, the patient must, of course, be billed.

Do not feel reticent to ask for payment. Patients know they must be charged for their visit. If the patient says, "I haven't that much money with me today," you can respond with "Oh, that's all right. We accept partial payments." In that way at least part of the fee is paid, and the patient is aware of his or her obligation.

Some dentists prefer to have the secretary present a bill at that time, accompanied by a stamped, addressed envelope. In that case you would say, "Mr. X, here is an addressed envelope that requires no postage. You can just put your check in here and mail it back to us."

Other dentists send monthly statements; this is a matter of office policy. Some are using computerized systems to do their billing.

When a patient has had extensive work, the bill may be a large one. It is best to make arrangements for partial payments over the period of time that the patient is being treated. To do this, discuss the arrangements for payment with the patient at the beginning of the treatment, or on the second visit if the patient appears upset at the first session.

For example you might say, "Mrs. J., Dr. X has explained to you that it will require six visits to complete your work. The fee will be $x. You don't need to pay the entire amount in one payment unless you wish to. However, we should make some arrangement about how the account is to be taken care of. Perhaps you would like to discuss this matter with your family, and talk to me again when you come in for your next treatment."

When the patient returns, try your best to arrange some definite weekly or monthly payment so that the total charge is covered by the end of the treatment period, if possible.

In certain offices fees are mentioned at the time the appointment is made, rather than after the visit; this depends of course, on the doctor.

Some dentists require the patient to make a payment before lab work is done. Here the office manager points out very matter-of-factly, "It is office policy that part of your bill be paid in advance." If this statement is questioned, the reply should be, "This policy has been arrived at after careful consideration, and I must abide by it." This statement should be made *pleasantly*, with a smile.

Whenever a patient questions a procedure, the same reply may be made. (For overdue fees, see "Collection Letters.")

You must bear in mind that your salary is paid out of monies received by your employer—if he or she is not paid, there may be no money to pay you.

Collection by attorneys or agencies. It is preferable to collect outstanding accounts through letters and telephone calls rather than through the services of attorneys or agencies. These services considerably decrease the funds which the doctor finally receives.

The choice of collection service may be turned over to you, but generally the doctor decides on the attorney or agency that will collect outstanding debts. If you are asked to decide, check with the local branch of the American Dental Association for a recommendation.

An attorney will almost unfailingly try to collect a bill without instituting suit against the patient, since such litigation is costly.

Should you choose an agency, be sure it is one that specializes in collecting debts owed to doctors. The techniques used are considerably different from those used by businesses.

Once a debt has been turned over to an outside party for collection, a portion of the money collected belongs to the collector. Even if the patient pays you, the attorney or the agency is entitled to the percentage previously agreed upon for collection.

It is absolutely essential that the doctor be informed, in advance, by either the attorney or the agency of the amount or percentage he or she will be charged. There have been cases in which attorneys have made settlements, after numerous negotiations, and have charged fees which were 100 percent of the settlement. The dentist actually received nothing! It is for this reason that financial arrangements must be made by you or by the doctor, and they should be in writing.

Collection letters.   The collection of outstanding bills is a very important part of the work of the office manager.

At the end of the month in which the patient was seen, and the bill incurred, a statement is sent. This statement may be a photocopy of his or her account, or a form letter used for the purpose. An envelope addressed to the doctor may be sent along with the statement. Sending an envelope facilitates payment, and some patients utilize it. The date of this statement is indicated on the patient's financial record.

At the end of the second month, another statement should be sent to the patient. On it write the words, "Please note: Second statement," or "Please note: Account overdue." An envelope should accompany this statement. Again the date should be recorded on the patient's record.

Discuss with your doctor whether or not to add a sentence such as the following: "If there is a problem regarding payment, please telephone us so that we can establish a plan

40

which would benefit both of us." He or she may wish to utilize this technique, which can result in partial payments.

If the patient does not respond to the second statement, it is time to begin Delinquent Account Collection Steps (DACS).

DAC Step I: Send a third statement. Accompanying the third statement should be a letter such as the following:

> Dear Mr. X:
> We have sent you two previous statements which you may have overlooked. These were dated _____ and _____ . Therefore your bill is now more than two months overdue. May we have your check by return mail. Thank you.
>
> Sincerely,
>
> _____
> Office Manager

Instead of a letter, you may enclose, with the statement, an impersonal, printed reminder, stating: "Please note: The attached statement indicates your account is well overdue. Please send your check. Thank you."

This type of reminder, because it is impersonal, may prove to be better as far as the patient's feelings are concerned. It is obvious, since the message has been printed, others are delinquent as well as the recipient.

DAC Step II: If, after three weeks to one month, you get no response, your follow-up procedure should be a telephone call to the patient.

Be sure you telephone while there are no other patients within hearing distance. Your call should be to the patient's home, rather than his or her place of business. When you telephone do the following:

1. State who you are. ("I'm Mary Ellen XYZ, Doctor R's office manager.")
2. Say, "We have sent you several statements of your account. Have you received them?"
3. Ask "Is there any problem?"

41

4. Ask "Can we arrange for you to pay some part of your bill each week?"
5. Say, "We will send you several envelopes. Please use these as reminders."

The sentences above are a skeletal outline. Add your own comments. Remember, never sound hostile or angry. Be sincere. Perhaps there is a problem. Make whatever arrangements that are necessary, so that some part of the bill is paid. Try to engage the patient in conversation—and do not take "No" for an answer—unless you absolutely must. Several calls, spaced two weeks apart, may be made if necessary.

DAC Step III: Send a Registered Letter. This letter must be very strong, without being angry. It should be sent by registered mail, return receipt requested.

In this letter, write:

Dear Mr. X:

"Your account is now very seriously overdue. Your bill, for _____ was incurred last _____.

We have notified you numerous times but you have failed to respond. We will therefore be forced to turn this bill over to our attorneys for collection unless payment is received by _____.

We hope it will not be necessary to take this action, but we will be forced to do so unless your account is cleared.

Very truly yours,

_____
Secretary to Dr._____

Keep careful notes of all collection steps taken. Note the action and the date. These notes are needed if the matter is turned over to another person or agency for collection. Speak to the doctor. Find out if he or she wishes to consult an agency or an attorney to collect this debt.

Collections—phone calls. You may find a telephone call can help you to collect from a patient who has ignored collection letters as well as bills.

When telephoning such "deadbeats," try the following:

Telephone the patient, and announce yourself in this manner: "Mr. Smith, this is Ms. Jones from Dr. Brown's office, calling." Then pause, and wait for the patient to reply. He or she will probably know exactly why you are calling and may respond, saying words to the effect, "I know my bill is overdue. I'm sending you a check." If that is the response, then you ask, "Can you give me a specific date, so that I'll be able to watch for your check in the mail?" If the patient, when answering the phone, says nothing, your next words should be, "Mr. Smith, there is an overdue balance of your bill of _____ dollars. (Fill in the specific amount.) I'm calling to try to make some specific arrangements with you, for payment. I know you're anxious to get the bill paid. How do you want to begin?" Be polite, but get specific answers, including dates of payment. Encourage the patient to pay even a small amount weekly.

If a person commits himself and then doesn't come through, it is time to take stronger action—such as turning the matter over to a collection agency.

It is important that your phone call is received by the person for whom it is intended. Try to call him or her at home, but if it's impossible to reach him or her, then call his or her place of work. In that case, however, if you cannot reach the patient, be careful when leaving a message to avoid any mention of the purpose of your call. Your message should be, "Mr. Smith, please call Ms. Jones of Dr. Brown's office."

Try in every way possible not to alienate the patient. If he or she becomes irritated or abusive, the best statement to make is, "I'm sure you realize my making this call is office procedure. You must know I am in charge of financial arrangements, and I have to clear accounts. I'd really appreciate your cooperation." In this way you make the matter as businesslike as you can.

Computerizing your office. The subject of computerization is a highly complex one. The information included here is very simple, but will give you some idea of what it is all about. Computers can do a great deal of work for you, with little effort. However, it is necessary to find the right setup for your office.

Computerizing your office

One of the most radical changes which you may make in your office is computerizing it. The first major decision is whether or not this should be done.

What Can a Computer Do For You? Here is a listing of some, but not all, of the functions which are possible:

It maintains your records alphabetically, by name, (or by number if you so desire).

It enters and retrieves information without your having to search files.

It is simple to update or correct records.

It provides patient recalls.

It duplicates records easily.

It prints and processes insurance forms and preauthorizations. When necessary, these may be duplicated easily.

It separates patient charges from estimated insurance payments.

It prints and processes patient statements with messages for overdue accounts.

It provides you with a listing of overdue accounts.

It provides forms and statements before the patient leaves the office.

It handles multiple insurance carriers for each patient.

What Are the Parts of a Computer System? There are two essential areas, one called hardware, the other software.

The hardware consists of:

1. The central processing unit (CPU) which is really the brain of the computer, and does the actual processing of the information.

2. The keyboard, for entering the data, which is much like a standard typewriter.

3. The output devices: These are the screen or monitor, which allows you to read the data, or a printer, which puts the data into print. You would probably use both.

4. The storage devices, which are either floppy discs, hard discs or tapes.

The software consists of programs, which carry out the

specific functions necessary. For example, a program may enable you to fill out dental insurance forms. (There is one available for the Universal ADA Insurance Claim Form.) Programs are available commercially for thousands of subjects, among them those you will need to use if you computerize your office.

There are a large variety of computers on the market today, and the choice is up to your employer. We can suggest a relatively inexpensive way in which you can begin the process of computerization. **Andent, Inc.,** 1000 North Avenue, Waukegan, IL 60085 has a system for under $4,500 which uses an Apple II Plus computer, with many programs, including the software for a full Medical Billing System. Check with dealers for details.

Beware! Before buying any computer, locate the software first. This means locating programs for each of the functions you want the computer to perform, and making sure your computer can use each of these programs. One can purchase a very expensive computer, capable of all sorts of things, but if there is no software for it, the process of creating it yourself becomes a very difficult, expensive proposition.

Computer newsletter. **Snyder Felmeister and Company,** 383 North Kings Highway, Cherry Hill, NJ 08034 publishes a newsletter called *Focus on Dental Computers,* which will supply dental personnel with ideas on how to use the office computer to greatest advantage, new software available, and for those who have not yet purchased a computer system, or are unhappy with the present one, a review of new systems as they are developed.

Consent forms. Information regarding any patient should never be given to anyone without a permission slip signed by the patient—or, if a child—the parents or guardians. Furthermore, if you doubt in any way that the signature is genuine, it is advisable to check with the patient by telephone or letter before revealing any information at all.

Persons who might request information include insurance company representatives, attorneys or even nurses.

Continuing education

The signed consent may be given by the patient, a legally qualified representative such as a parent or guardian, an executor or administrator of an estate or an agency designated by the court as a guardian.

This consent must be directed to the doctor, and indicate to whom the information is to go. It should include what information is to be released, the period the patient was under the doctor's care, and should be dated after the patient was treated.

This consent is necessary when giving information to other doctors, schools, other institutions and insurance companies.

The following form may be used:

Dear Dr. ————————————

I hereby request that my records in regard to ——————————

————————————————————————————

————————————————————————————

be released, and sent to ——————————————————

at the following address ——————————————————

————————————
Patient's signature

Continuing education. Any courses you take that upgrade your skills are eminently worthwhile. These may involve any aspect of your work including public relations, psychology, technical work, office management, bookkeeping or filing systems, or the use of new products.

Your employer may be willing to pay for your courses. In the event that this is not the case, any money you expend is deductible from your income taxes. Courses taken for a new career are not deductible; they must be to improve your work in your present career.

Courses may be taken through the **Dental Society,**

through colleges or through adult-education programs available in your area.

It is entirely possible to discover you are familiar with much of the material covered. However, even if you pick up only one or two items, the course may prove to be worthwhile. All upgrading of your skills is important to you and your office.

Correspondence courses. The **ADAA** offers a number of correspondence courses (called "Continuing Education Courses") at nominal costs. The topics are very useful and supply valuable practical information. For example, topics such as "Introduction to Advanced Dental Practice Management," "Sharpening Curets and Sickle Scalers," "Introduction to Basic Pathology," and "The Construction of Temporary Acrylic Splints" are included.

Costs are reduced for members of the **ADAA.** For full information, contact the organization at 666 North Lake Shore Drive, Suite 1130, Chicago, IL 60611. Ask for a listing of all services offered by the ADAA. Then discuss these services with your employer. This is an excellent way to show your professionalism.

Cosmetic appeal. Your employer certainly does some dentistry for purely esthetic reasons, and all facets of dentistry have an esthetic aspect. You can play an import role in regard to this, by admiring the work your employer does.

It is important that you be sincere in your expression of admiration. You can ask patients, particularly women, to show you how they look when their dental work is completed. Then react with enthusiasm and pleasure.

Be careful not to use a "canned speech." One dental assistant commented, "That's the best work Dr. J. has ever done." The problem was she said this to everyone! (The word got around, and her comments were much more detrimental than helpful.)

Your teeth, too, should look their very best. They should be stain free, and can be made to appear brighter if you wear a red lipstick. (This can be recommended to patients if done diplomatically.)

Your employer may wish you to present samples of tooth paste to patients to keep their teeth as attractive as possible.

Your office must be well lit for your patients to look their best. Dim lights cause a dingy appearance.

If your employer uses some of the more modern techniques such as tooth bonding and acid-etched retained bridges, be sure you can explain these procedures to the patient in easily understandable terms, as well as stressing the conservative nature of these procedures, which do not involve injections or removal of sound tooth structure.

Credit extending. Many patients request they be billed for the doctor's services. Yet the question of whether or not the patient will promptly honor these bills is an important one.

You will already have had the patient fill out a Financial Record Form. There are certain additional questions you may ask which will give you an idea of the patient's ability to pay his or her bills. The following may be used:

1. How long have you lived in this community?
2. How long have you lived at your present address? (If less than one year, ask for the previous address.)
3. How long have you worked for your present employer? (You already know who that is from the Financial Record Form.)

From these few questions you can get an idea of the person's relative stability. Should a patient be hesitant about answering, or resistant, discuss this with the doctor. Decide with the doctor in advance how far you should go in your routine or special credit investigations.

Patient credit may be checked with a credit-reporting agency. When a substantial amount of money from a businessman or women is concerned, various agencies such as the Credit Bureau are available for consultation. Check the "Yellow Pages" for "Credit reporting agencies."

Once the patient has accepted the doctor's services, he or she has an obligation to pay the bill. Credit terms should be determined in advance—some doctors have arranged to accept Visa or Master card. It is the job of the office manager to collect as much of the doctor's money as possible, and to be sure patients understand the situation. However, this must be done in a pleasant, nonhostile way, using as much tact and diplomacy as possible.

Criminal actions. Each person is responsible, according to the law, for his or her own actions. In the event that you are asked to do something by your employer or a patient which you know to be illegal, or feel may possibly be, be aware that you will be considered either as the perpetrator or as an accessory, and may, consequently, get into serious legal difficulty. This is true in spite of the fact that you may have been instructed to do this deed by the dentist who is employing you. While you are expected to be loyal to your employer, you should not allow yourself to be placed in the position of committing an illegal act or acts.

You should also refrain from performing tasks that are outside the scope of your duties. You should not ever, for example, prescribe medication without the doctor's instructions.

Special care should be taken regarding the handling of narcotics. All drugs must be prescribed in writing using the special number assigned to the doctor. All prescription pads and particularly those bearing this number must be kept under lock and key.

Criticism, accepting. No one is perfect. In your role as either a dental auxiliary or an office manager, you are bound to make some mistakes, and someone, whether it be your doctor or a fellow staff member, is going to have to correct you. It is very important to your growth in your career that you learn to accept criticism graciously.

Do you get upset when you are told you made an error? If you do, try to figure out why. The chances are you feel the person correcting you is saying, "You are no good," or "You are stupid (or careless) for having done this." Actually that person is saying, "You made a mistake. Correct it," but you are taking the remark *personally.*

How do you feel when you must correct someone? You probably are not very happy doing so. The person correcting you often feels the same way, but it is very nonproductive to allow anyone to continue making mistakes time after time. If you can avoid getting upset, you can make the other person's life easier—and your own as well. If you are constantly on the defensive when you are corrected, if you sulk or withdraw, people will stop trying to correct you. There is always the danger they will get frustrated and react, later on, out of that frustration.

The simplest, most effective thing to do is to say, sincerely, "I'm sorry; I'll remember that in the future," and make as sure as you possibly can that you do remember it.

Sometimes, in the situation of being found to have made an error, a person will try to make explanations for it. "What happened was I . . ." Believe it or not, this does not prove to be as effective as the simpler remark given above.

If you find you make the same mistake over and over again, sit down and try to figure out why you do so. What is causing this error? Are you trying to work too quickly? Are you not paying attention? Have you not learned the correct procedure? Are you being interrupted too often? Whatever the reason is, uncovering it should make it possible for you to remedy the situation.

It should be noted here that correcting another's error should *never* be done in front of a patient. If circumstances require this, however, it must be accomplished as diplomatically as possible. The image of a quarreling office is a sure detriment to any practice.

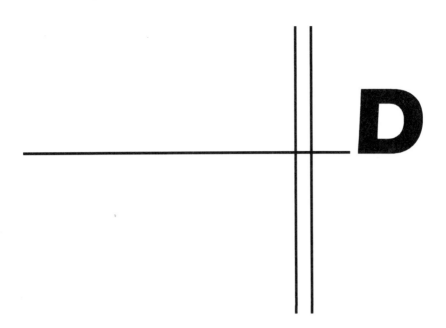

Day sheet. The day sheet lists the names of the patients the doctor is scheduled to see during the day and the time of their appointments. It is written up by the person in charge of the appointment book at the same time she arranges the appointments.

If the doctor has more than one treatment room, a copy of the day sheet should be placed in each room.

This sheet should be written so that the doctor has no difficulty in reading it. In addition to the patient's name, the doctor may wish to have indicated on it the nature of the visit as well.

When an appointment is cancelled, the name should be crossed off the day sheet, and replaced by the name of the person filling in.

Deaf patients. Because it may not be obvious that a patient is deaf, if you encounter someone who seems to have trouble hearing you, ask him a question in a low voice while looking down. If there is no response, raise your voice, and repeat the question. If the patient is able to hear this, then you should speak in that tone of voice. If not, then assume the patient has a problem. Speak slowly, loudly and distinctly so that if the patient lip reads, he can understand you.

However, when giving instructions, write them—and have the patient read them aloud—so that you are sure they are understood.

If the doctor does not use a printed questionnaire, prepare one. This makes it possible to be sure the patient is not confused. Ask such questions as the following:

1. Why are you seeing the doctor?
2. When did the problem begin?
3. Do you have pain? Where?
4. What other symptoms do you have?
5. Is the pain sharp or dull? (Cross out the one which *does not* describe your condition.)
6. Is the pain constant or intermittent?
7. Do you take any medication? If so, what?
8. Do you have any other health problems? If so, what?
9. How long have you had it?
10. Who is the doctor treating you for it?

Decorating the office. The waiting room of your office should be as bright and cheerful as possible. It should be well lit by table lamps, which are the most pleasant and flattering form of lighting.

Walls should be done in a warm color such as a light yellow, rather than a flat white.

Pictures of all types should be placed on the walls. Many patients enjoy seeing photographs of the doctor's family, or of things which interest him or her.

The furniture should be of practical covering, but of pleasant colors rather than dark brown or black. The same is true of the floor covering. A color scheme of yellow, deep orange or rust, with light brown and/or green can be very effective.

Many people prefer chairs to couches, so that a waiting room may be done entirely in chairs, or with one couch. Coverings should be chosen which are durable. Vinyls are good, as are tweeds.

The furnishings should be replaced when they become shabby, and the office repainted every two years—or sooner if it becomes necessary.

Dental assistant—general considerations. The dental assistant has specific duties which must be accomplished for optimum efficiency in the office. The dental assistant's primary function is to aid the dentist in all procedures requiring "four hands." Four-handed dentistry came about with the development of the high-speed drill, which requires a copious water spray that must be evacuated continuously from the patient's mouth. Also, since the drill revolves at speeds up to 300,000 rpm, protection of the cheeks, gums and tongue is a necessity. Suctioning of water and saliva and retraction of oral soft tissues led to the development of four-handed dentistry, which became the first priority for the assistant in the dentistry of today.

The other major task given the dental assistant is to maintain the equipment and inventory of the office. Maintenance includes general cleaning of all surfaces of the operatory, being responsible for the sterilization of all instruments, and insuring that all necessary supplies are on hand.

The specific limits of what chairside duties the dental assistant is able to perform varies from state to state; your employer will be the arbiter of the duties you can perform. The more tasks that the dental assistant can legally do, the less time the dentist must spend with the patient, and the more efficient and profitable the practice will be.

The following are some of the basic tasks which the dental assistant is called upon to perform:

1. Prepare the operatory for each patient.
2. Supply necessary instruments and equipment.
3. Pull files of patients listed on the day sheet.
4. Prepare patients for examination, including, if so requested, the medical history and vital signs.
5. Assist doctor during examinations and during all procedures, including charting, and taking and developing x-ray and study models.
6. Care for instruments.

7. Keep an inventory of supplies.

8. Order supplies when necessary.

9. Enter information on patient's charts.

Each of these duties are discussed further in this book.

Dental hygienist, career information. Dental Hygiene was originated in 1913 by Dr. Alfred Fones, to provide education and preventive oral treatments for school children. Today, Dental Hygiene is defined by the **American Dental Hygienists Association House of Delegates** as "the health profession which in cooperation with the dental profession provides services to promote optimal oral health care for the public."

State laws govern the types of settings in which a hygienist may work, but they generally include dental offices and other facilities employing a dentist or having dental supervision. Many school systems and public agencies also employ program graduates.

Dental Hygiene functions vary depending on individual state dental-practice acts, but traditionally the dental hygienist will:

1. Collect patient data to compile a medical and dental history.

2. Perform diagnostic tests.

3. Examine hard and soft tissues of the head and the neck region (including an oral cancer exam).

4. Instruct patients in home-care procedures (to maintain a healthy oral environment).

5. Expose and process radiographs.

6. Assist patients with dietary analysis and nutritional counseling.

7. Apply caries-preventive agents.

8. Remove hard and soft deposits from the teeth.

9. Provide supportive treatment services under the direction of a dentist.

10. Design and implement community and school health programs.

In some states, a dental hygienist may:

1. Place and remove temporary fillings and periodontal dressings.
2. Polish and recontour defective restorations.
3. Administer local anesthesia and nitrous oxide.
4. Perform gingival curettage.
5. Place and carve amalgam and tooth-colored restorations.

Education. Dental Hygiene is a licensed profession; to be eligible for licensure, a candidate must complete a minimum educational requirement of at least two years of college in an accredited Dental Hygiene Program. Programs are found in community colleges, dental schools, colleges and universities, and technical institutes. (A complete listing of accredited programs throughout the country can be obtained from the **American Dental Association Commission on Dental Accreditation.**)

Selection of a program may depend on your career goals, financial considerations or geographic location. Two years in an Associate Degree or Certificate Program will prepare you as a clinical practitioner. Some students select a Baccalaureate Program with a major in Dental Hygiene; others choose to major in education, psychology, business or health administration, which broadens their background, allowing access to other areas of practice. A Master's Degree in Dental Hygiene or a related area can provide additional concentrated study and preparation.

It is very important that one contact the program one is interested in at least a full year prior to the desired admission date (nearly always a Fall Semester) for an application and specific admission requirements.

Licensure. Following graduation from an accredited program, the dental hygienist is eligible to take the written National Board Examination and a state or regional examination (practical/clinical.) The candidate must pass both the written and practical/clinical examinations and be licensed by the State

Board of Dental Examiners in the state(s) selected for practice. Most jurisdictions accept the National Board Examination; those who do not provide their own written examination. Until recently, dental hygienists had to take a practical/clinical examination for each state they wanted to practice in. The establishment of Regional Examining Boards, to which a group of states subscribe and accept test results, has greatly reduced the time and expense involved in hygienist's moving across state lines. Most states also require passing a written test on the State Dental Practice Act. The rapid growth in scope of Dental Hygiene has prompted some states to require that candidates be tested in certain expanded functions and that a certain number of continuing-education credits be earned yearly to maintain licensure. (Current information on licensure is available from the **American Association of Dental Examiners.**)

Dental specialties.   It is important for all office personnel to be familiar with the dental specialties. They are arranged here alphabetically.

Endodontist.   A specialist who diagnoses and treats diseases of the pulp and periapical area of the teeth. The most frequently performed service the endodontist renders is root canal therapy. Often, they receive referrals from general dentists when the tooth needing treatment has curved roots, or small or partially calcified root canals.

Oral Surgeon.   A specialist who diagnoses and treats diseases of the jaws and surrounding structures. Surgeons are trained to set fractures of the jaws, remove tumors and other growths, and extract impacted teeth. Many surgeons are affiliated with, and competent to admit patients to, a hospital, and have the training necessary to use general anesthesia or intravenous sedation when performing various procedures.

Orthodontist.   A dentist who diagnoses and treats the developing teeth and bones of the oral cavity to insure healthy occlusion. The orthodontist examines and surveys the deciduous, mixed or adult dentition (often with panoramic x-rays), and uses corrective bands and wires to shift out-of-place teeth into

56

healthy relationships. He may also recommend the selective extraction of teeth when it is necessary.

Pedodontist. A dentist who specializes in treating children. Although there is little difference in procedures performed on adults and children, it is often easier and more economical for the general dentist to refer very young or apprehensive children to the pedodontist.

Periodontist. A dentist who specializes in the diagnosis and treatment of the gums and bones supporting the teeth. Often, patients are referred to the periodontist for treatment where severe neglect of oral hygiene has created conditions requiring surgical intervention to prevent early loss of teeth.

Prosthodontist. A dentist who specializes in diagnoses and treatment of premature loss of the dentition. Often, patients are referred to the prosthodontist when they have trouble tolerating a prosthesis fabricated by the general dentist, or when preexisting conditions are such that the dentist sees problems ahead.

Dentistry, history of. Dentistry, as a profession, is comparatively young, having come into its own in the middle 1700s, through the work of the man often called the "Founder of Modern Dentistry," Pierre Fauchard. (Medicine on the other hand, goes back thousands of years to the time Hippocrates wrote his famous oath.)

However, the need for dental care was recognized very early in the history of man. The ancients, who believed in evil spirits, attributed toothaches to their handiwork. Priests were the people whose task it was to drive off these spirits, often doing so with chants and herbs. As long as the spirit world was the basis of religious belief, dental pain was explained in that way.

Evidence has been found proving that the Phoenicians and Egyptians began doing a very early type of prosthetic work. They used gold wire to tighten loose teeth by binding them together, and also used animal teeth to replace human teeth. The Greeks are believed to have used chalk to clean the teeth, and had a type of instrument to do extractions.

Other early civilizations made contributions as well. The Israelites used salt water for cleaning, and the Koran actually describes a primitive type of toothbrush and toothpaste.

Even today the people of the Masai tribe in East Africa use twigs to clean their teeth—using them in exactly the manner we use such equipment as *Stimu-dents* today.

By the year 500 B.C., people were sharing their problems, and different remedies were tried. The ones that proved worthwhile were recorded, and thus it became possible to transmit knowledge. The barbers of the time took on the added function of caring for teeth—and became known as "Barber-Surgeons." (They were also called Treaters of Teeth or Tooth Operators.) It was these people who did the extractions, and were in charge of dental care for hundreds of years.

In the Middle Ages, in Europe, monks were the dental practitioners, until 1131 when the clergy was forbidden from performing any surgical procedures. It was then that barber-surgeons took over, and remained in charge until the 19th century.

However, in France, Pierre Fauchard published *The Surgeon Dentist* in 1728, in which he covered dental anatomy, tooth decay, dental surgery, gum disease and the use of medications. Fauchard's influence was great—more books were published, and instruments developed to improve techniques.

The development of dentistry in colonial America came directly from France. Two French dentists came to teach the men in the colonial army.

Paul Revere advertised, he "still continues the business of a dentist, and flatters himself that from the experiences he has had these two years (in which time he has fixt some hundreds of teeth) that he can fix them as well as any Surgeon Dentist who ever came from London. He fixes them in such a manner that they are not only an ornament but of real use in speaking and eating. He cleans the teeth and will wait on any gentleman or lady at their lodging." This advertisement appeared in the Boston Gazette in 1770. Revere was renowned as a silversmith, and also worked in gold and did engraving.

George Washington had dentures, examples of which are in the Smithsonian, being on loan from the Baltimore College of Dental Surgery, University of Maryland. They were made by John Greenwood from ivory, and were secured in the mouth by spiral springs of gold.

In 1791 the first dental clinic to treat the poor opened in New York City, but throughout early United States history most dentistry was practiced by barbers and other people not trained in the field.

It was in the 19th century that dentistry became a profession. Many tech nical advances were made, including the use of vulcanite rubber denture base in 1854, and in 1895 the use of silver amalgam for fillings.

It was in the 19th century, too, that anesthesia was developed. In the 1840's nitrous oxide and ether were introduced, the former in 1844, and the latter in 1846.

In order for dentistry to become a profession, dental schools had to be established. The first was the Baltimore College of Dental Surgery. However, it was not until after the Civil War that there was a small public demand for dental school graduates. By 1870 there were 10,000 practicing dentists, but only 1,000 were graduates of dental schools. By 1960 there were 87 dental colleges in the United States.

The world's first dental association, the American Society of Dental Surgeons was established in the United States in 1840. The first American textbook on dentistry had been published in 1801.

Dentistry continued to progress in many areas, including instrumentation, dental technologies, oral hygiene, preventive dentistry and the education of dentists.

Until 1869, a dental course consisted of 16 weeks (one year) of training, with no predental requirements. From 1870-91, two academic years, or 16-20 weeks, were required. Fom 1891 to 1917 dental courses were lengthened to three academic years (28 to 32 weeks each). Between 1899 and 1902 one year of high school was required; from 1902 to 1907 two years, and from 1907 to 1910 three years of high school. In 1910 high school graduation was required; in 1921 two years of college. Today preference is given to college graduates, although three years is the minumum to fulfill the requirements. In 1917 the dental course was increased to four years of 32 weeks each year. Predental college requirements include courses in biology, physics and chemistry.

With the introduction of the four-year program dental education reached the truly professional level of today. There are more than 126,000 dentists in the United States today, 90 percent of whom are in private practice. A license is necessary in every state.

Desk work space. When you must do desk work for a large proportion of your time, it is important that you arrange your desk in such a fashion that you do not have to place undue strain on your body. Here are some tips in that regard.

1. Be sure you do not have to stretch or twist your body to answer the telephone, to write in your appointment book or to type.
2. Everything you use frequently should be within arm's length.
3. Clear the desk space of things which you do not use frequently. These can be placed in drawers or out of the way, but they should not clutter up your work space and prevent you from reaching the things you use often.
4. Keep the supplies you use, such as forms, typing paper, etc. in drawers close to your work area.
5. Arrange your drawers so that they contain materials you use frequently. Find a place to store other things so that they do not take up space—or require your taking time to reach the essentials.
6. Be sure you have enough light to enable you to see without squinting. The light should not shine into your eyes, however, but be shaded to protect you.

These tips are meant to help you become more efficient.

Detail men or women. The detail man or woman is employed by a pharmaceutical (drug) company. It is his or her function to present information to the dentist regarding products which his or her company markets. The purpose of this is so that the doctor will prescribe that company's drugs.

Often the detail men or women will present the doctor with samples of not only new products but also other products manufactured by their employer.

You and your employer should arrive at a policy regarding detail people. It may be that the doctor wll see them if he or she can spare the time. However this should be worked out beforehand so that you will know how to proceed when the situation occurs.

If it is inconvenient for the doctor to see the detail person at the time of his or her visit, you may schedule an appointment (if this is office policy). It is to the detail person's advantage to see the doctor when he or she is not rushed or distracted. It is to the doctor's advantage to get the information detail people can give him or her. However, make sure the doctor is reminded at the end of a designated period of time. In this way he or she can terminate the discussion or prolong it at his discretion.

The detail person should be notified if the doctor is unable to keep an appointment.

Most detail people are well spoken and courteous. If you find they are not, you may wish to notify the Personnel Director of the company they represent.

Diabetic dental patients, how to handle. Diabetes is a common disease—there are an estimated ten million people, of all ages, who have it. They are affected dentally, because of the delay in the healing time which they experience. They also have a decreased resistance to periodontal disease and to infection.

If your employer is treating diabetic patients, and you would be aware of this from their medical history, it is advisable to have a sugar source available, should the patient need some immediately. Orange juice is such a source.

The healing process should be carefully watched, and the patient should be seen several times for this purpose. He or she should also be given very precise instructions for dental care.

It is necessary, too, to check the medications the diabetic patient is taking, because of possible drug interaction. Make

Dictation

the doctor aware of these by attaching a note, written in red, to the patient's chart, just as is done with all serious illnesses. Your doctor may wish to check with the patient's physician, and his or her name should be available.

Should your practice have many diabetic patients, see the article by Zoeller, G.N., and Kadis, B. in *General Dentist,* 29(1): 58-61, 1981.

Dictation. Doctors give dictation when they fill out reports, write letters or fill out records. If this is your situation, make sure your work is accurate when transcribing. An error can be very harmful; therefore if you have any questions whatsoever review them with your doctor.

Try to do your transcribing during a time when your telephone is least busy.

Have all material to be sent out checked by the doctor, unless you are instructed to do otherwise.

Diplomacy. The dental secretary or assistant is often in a position to act as a peacemaker when a patient is upset or in distress. This is especially true when the patient is upset with the doctor. Perhaps the doctor has been called to an emergency and the waiting room is filled with patients. By apologizing for the delay quietly but sincerely, patients can be made to understand the situation. If a patient is highly excitable or overwrought, quiet words of support can make a great deal of difference.

Patients at times become upset about bills. Here, too, quiet reasoning and reassurance are necessary.

You must consider each patient with a problem individually. When a patient talks about a lawsuit, you must follow the procedures mentioned above. Do not allow yourself to be threatened by this word. Instead be supportive and understanding. You may use the technique of repeating the patient's words, after prefacing them with "I understand." For example, "I understand you're upset. Please try to be patient. I'll try to arrange for the doctor to see you as soon as possible." This technique of repeating the patient's complaints in their own words is called "active listening," and may be a great help in communicating in many situations.

Disappearing patients. In many dental practices there are patients who have not paid their bills, who disappear, and who "skip" town. Should you have any, there are certain procedures which may be of use to you.

1. If a letter is returned to you, check the address. Many times letters are sent back because the address was copied incorrectly.

2. Call the patient at his residence. If he cannot be reached, call the telephone "information operator," and ask for the new number. If you are told it is *unlisted,* at least you know the patient is still in your community.
   Next call his or her number at work. Do not reveal any information but leave a message asking him or her to call you at your number. "Please phone Mrs. Blue at 987-6543." *Not,* "Please call Dr. Brown's office."

3. If you are still unsuccessful, check with the Motor Vehicle Bureau.

4. Another possibility, if the patient gave references, is to contact them. Leave the same type of message as Item 2 above.

5. If the patient has children, a check with the school they attended may reveal a new address.

6. If the amount owed is sizeable, ask your employer if he or she wishes the account turned over to an agency for collection. Your knowledge of the patient's circumstances can help in making this decision.

Distributing printed materials. For patient education, your doctor may wish to distribute printed materials relevant to his or her specialty. These are often available from the American Dental Association.

Before giving any material away, your doctor should check it carefully to be sure it does not contain any information contrary to his or her views.

Private companies, such as the pharmaceutical manufacturers, also supply printed materials for distribution to pa-

Doctor signed letters and reports

tients. These, however, may contain advertising material, and should be checked carefully by the doctor before distributing them.

Doctor signed letters and reports. All letters and reports should be checked by the doctor. It is far too easy for errors to be made, particularly when the doctor has used unfamiliar terminology. Before any material of a technical nature goes out, the doctor should review and sign it. Check your spelling in Section II of this book, or, if necessary, in a dictionary.

Copies of all letters and reports should be kept on file. If the correspondence is in regard to a patient, it should be put in his or her file.

If otherwise, it should be kept in the file under "Correspondence."

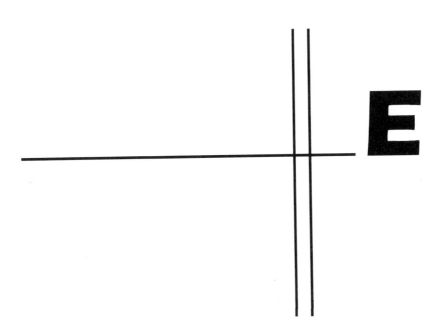

Elderly patients. It is a fact that people are living longer today than they ever did before. However, they are, for the most part, not in perfect dental health. In a dentist's office you will probably see many more than the percentage in the population at large.

Many of the elderly develop what seem to be paranoid tendencies. A good many feel unwanted and unloved, and need support and affection. If you can offer a little of each you can help them, and as a result be of genuine value to your employer.

Address each person by name. Never, ever, call someone "Pop" or "Grandma"—even if you are well aware they can rightfully be addressed in this manner. "Mr. Jones" or "Mrs. Smith" is correct.

It is wise to ask the person, speaking in a relatively soft voice, "Can you hear me?" Then, judge from the loudness of the reply at what level you must speak. If there is a hearing problem, speak slowly and distinctly, but even then do not shout. Look at the person as you speak to him or her.

Be careful not to behave in a manner which might be interpreted as patronizing. Elderly patients may, and often do have forms which have to be filled out. Do this pleasantly and willingly.

Old people are forgetful and may not have all of the information you need. With this in mind, request they return to you with the necessary documentation, but don't show anger or annoyance.

If the patient appears to be slightly infirm, help him or her when necessary.

If any instructions are given to the patient make sure he or she can read them. If not, type or print them on a sheet of paper which can be easily read. If they are complicated, it is essential you break them down into steps the patient easily understands.

Be reassuring in your manner. Many many times the reassurance is a very important part of the treatment. For example, patients may come into the office and say to you words to the effect, "My back is very bad today," or "My arthritis is killing me." If you reply, "Mrs. Smith, the weather is changing, I think. The doctor will see you in a few minutes." That seems to make people feel better. You can diffuse a lot of anxiety and resentment in this way, and help make the visit a better experience.

A fall can be a very serious thing for an older person, since many break bones rather easily. Therefore, make sure the floors are not slippery, and there is nothing for the patient to stumble over.

If the patient has a heart condition, or any other medical problem and is under treatment by a physician, you must check with his or her office to find out if there are any specific instructions for your doctor. Often, your employer will insist on speaking to the physician himself.

Emergencies Discuss with your employer how he or she wishes you to handle emergencies, since some must be handled immediately while others require only a telephone call to a pharmacist. It is best to establish standard policy and procedures that you are to follow.

Any emergency should take precedence over routine procedures. Arrange for the patient to either speak to the doctor or come into the office. Have an operatory available, should the patient be coming to the office.

Write out, with the doctor, a list of the information which you must obtain either from the patient or a person accompanying him or her.

Often a telephone call by the doctor prescribing medication will suffice. If an office visit is indicated, a good rule of thumb is to verbally question the patient as to his medical history, even after he or she has filled out a medical questionnaire. A good technique is the I.B.M. rule—that is:

(I)llness—any illness requiring hospitalization within the last two years?

(B)leeding—any bleeding problems associated with routine cuts or bruises or previous dental extractions?

(M)edication—any medication being taken now?

Find out from your doctor if he feels it is his job to ask these questions. It is far better to be on the side of caution than to be negligent.

Ethics. It is important that you as a dental auxiliary realize you should never give advice regarding dental problems. While it may be very tempting at times, it is dangerous to do so. When you are asked questions, it is a far better idea to say "I think you'd better check with the doctor", or " . . . with your doctor." Friends and relatives often do ask for advice, which you are not really qualified to give. Furthermore, you do not have all of the information the doctor has. Telling a patient to take a certain drug, for example, may be very dangerous because you are not familiar with his or her medical conditions or history.

Never criticize work done by any dentist (certainly, most of all, by your employer). You don't know what the condition of that patient's mouth was, or what the goal of treatment was. (Possibly the patient had told the doctor to keep costs down to a minimum.)

Exercises for the busy assistant

Should you offer the wrong information, it is possible you might be sued or even lose your own job.

Never gossip about anything related to patients, your employer or other dentists since there is no way in which you could benefit from it.

If a person has a dental problem, encourage him or her to seek appropriate dental care. In this way you are acting in a completely professional manner.

Exercises for the busy assistant. You need exercise to keep your stress level down, and to make you more limber. One of the best is for you to take a brisk walk during your lunch hour.

In the office you can do the following:

1. Reach up with one hand, and hold that position for about 15 seconds. (To count seconds, count locomotive one, locomotive two, and so on. Or you may use one-thousand-one, one-thousand-two, etc.) Then repeat with the other hand.

2. While sitting at your desk, you can do an excellent exercise. Push back your chair, and then, while sitting in it, reach with both hands behind the back of the chair. Clasp your hands, and then lean your body forward, pulling down your shoulders as you do so.

3. While sitting, pull your stomach muscles in, and hold for six seconds. Relax, and repeat several times. Or you may raise your feet off the floor several inches and rotate them.

4. You can also rotate your head, and raise and lower your shoulders.

All of these exercises will help you to avoid the fatigue caused by remaining seated at your desk most of the day.

Expenditures, book of. This record should be kept by the office manager. It indicates all monies paid out in the form of cash or checks. It takes into consideration:

1. How much was paid out.

2. The form of payment. If a check was used, the number of the check should be indicated.

3. The nature of the expense. This would include any and all business deductions such as:

Rent	Taxes
Electric	Insurance
Telephone	Interest or bank charges
Office Salaries	Laundry
Supplies	Cleaning services
Drugs	Entertainment
Equipment purchased	Accounting services
Equipment repair	Postage
Laboratory fees and expenses	Miscellaneous
Automobile expenses	

The ledger selected for this should have adequate columns to indicate those expenses which come up most frequently. It is very valuable because it shows the doctor, very quickly, where his or her money goes.

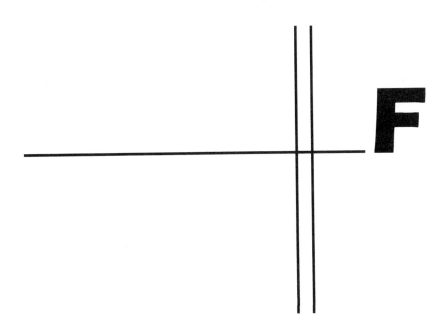

Fainting.   Before a patient faints, they will exhibit premonitory signs. The person feels uncomfortable, weak, squeamish and giddy, and begins to sweat. If unrelieved, the condition worsens and the patient faints. He or she becomes pale, sweats, and has a thin, rapid pulse that slows down. Then there is a fall in blood pressure and a loss of consciousness. If the patient remains in a faint for more than a few minutes, muscular contractions may occur, and the patient may wet or soil himself or herself.

In the premonitory state, it may be adequate to have the patient lie or sit down and lower the head between the knees for a minute or two until the feeling passes.

If the patient is unconscious, he or she should be placed lying down, with the feet slightly elevated. Clothing should be loosened. For any fainting episode, notify the doctor immediately. If the doctor is not in the office, call an ambulance.

A mild stimulant, such as ammonia (inhaled) or cold water (applied to the face) may be used.

If a patient faints while in the waiting room before treatment, notify your doctor immediately.

Fainting is also called syncope.

Family or marital problems.   Be extremely careful never to become involved in family or marital problems. Patients often are upset and need to talk about things that are bothering them. Yet, as a dental auxiliary or office manager, you cannot spare the time to listen to them. Nor is it your function to do so.

If you find you are faced with this problem frequently, you may ask your employer if he or she will allow you to recommend a mental health facility, or possibly other professionals such as psychiatrists or social workers.

It is dangerous to offer advice because then you may be blamed if things do not work out well. It is very risky for anyone to advise others in the space of a few minutes because one cannot possibly have all of the facts. This is why professionals require several hours of interviewing before they begin to advise or counsel.

This surely does not mean you are to be abrupt or brush the patient off. It requires you to tactfully remove yourself from the situation with words to the effect, "Please excuse me. Doctor needs me in the treatment room."

In one case, however, you would probably have to function differently. In the case of child abuse, check with your state **Association for the Prevention of Cruelty to Children.** You may be mandated to report this type of situation to them.

Women who have been abused should be advised to contact the police department.

Fee schedules.   Since you will be in charge of fee collection it is important that you understand fully the doctor's fee schedule. Never assume anything. Discuss the basic fees charged by your employer with him or her, and then determine how you will be notified of any variation in it.

Since many doctors vary their fees on occasion it is important that you set up a direct line of communication.

Files; business, active.   All matters related to the office are kept in this file. Material is filed according to subjects. The following listing may be used as a basis:

Bills	Equipment
Correspondence	Insurance

Dental Associations   Supplies, dental

Medications   Supplies, office

Printed materials   Taxes

This file is particularly valuable when tax returns are being prepared. It must be kept up-to-date, and every piece of relevant material should be placed in it for future reference.

Your employer may wish to include his or her personal papers in this file. In that case prepare a separate set of folders, with the items listed above. Use a different colored label for these, so that they are not mistaken for regular business folders. These files are totally separate from the patient files.

Files; inactive. Patients' files: Folders of patients no longer being seen by the doctor should be removed from the active file and placed in another filing cabinet, for storage. However, this cabinet should be placed in an accessible spot, so that the folders, when needed, may be located easily.

Business files: Folders should be used to store materials which may subsequently be needed. The materials should be kept in the inactive file until the statute of limitations runs out. This varies from state to state.

Never clean out these files without discussing their contents with your employer. Certain papers may be needed after long periods of time.

Files, patient, active. Each folder should be labeled with the following information:

Patient's name; family name first

Address

Social Security number

Date of birth

Telephone number (home)

Telephone number (business)

Parents' names should be indicated on children's folders. When the address is different from that of the child (as in the case of remarriage) that should be indicated as well.

Filing tips

Folders of all patients currently being seen, and those who were seen within the last three years should be kept in the active file. Your employer may decide to change that time span, depending on the nature of his or her practice.

Files should be kept in alphabetical order. Indicators should be used to separate letters.

In some offices, doctors prefer to file the records of all of the members of a family in the same folder. If this system is used, the following information should appear on the front of the folder.

Family name (typed in capital letters and underlined)

Names of the family members

Address of the family

Social Security number (of the parent)

Birth dates

Telephone number (home)

Telephone number (business) of the parent

Filing tips.

1. Establish your files to leave room for future expansion.

2. Do not pack drawers too tightly. Leave four to six inches of working-and-expansion space for better visibility and ease of working.

3. Do not overload folders. Transfer material which is not current.

4. Be sure every piece of material filed is necessary. Do not, for example, file letters in envelopes.

5. Insert a card whenever you remove a folder. This saves time when replacing it.

6. Make sure the name is printed very clearly.

7. Where names are similar, use first and middle names for easy identification.

8. If the bottom drawer of your filing cabinet is empty be sure to place heavy books in it to prevent its falling over. Do not take a chance on being hurt.

74

Filling in for absent staff members. It is necessary for each staff member to perform the most important tasks of the others, so that in the event of a staff member being ill, the critical tasks get done.

If there are part-time employees, they should be trained as understudies for the principal employees of the office. When one person is designated as office manager, one of her tasks must be to supervise coverage when necessary.

Tasks which can wait do not have to be done by the person filling in unless the absent person will be out for a period of time exceeding one week.

The *Procedures Manual* is especially useful in this regard.

Financial arrangements. Although it is the dentist who makes the decisions regarding payments, it is the dental assistant who actually deals with the patients in financial terms.

Your employer will establish a fee schedule, and a variety of payment plans with you. You must fully understand every aspect of every plan before you use them in dealing with any patients.

It is absolutely essential that you be as tactful and understanding as possible when dealing with financial arrangements. Avoid making any comments which might cause embarrassment to a patient. Be careful that you do not imply that a patient who pays his bill in cash is preferable to one who does not elect that payment plan.

At the same time, be businesslike though friendly. If you are not serious, patients may get the idea that they can be lax or delinquent when it comes to paying their bills. Set up a plan which they can live with comfortably.

There are, of course, a number of plans which may be utilized. The following arrangements are available to the patient:

Cash—Payment in full on day patient is treated. Some dentists offer a discount of from two to five percent because bills need not be sent.

Credit Cards—One of the most frequent means of transacting business today. May be used effectively in a dental office.

Financial arrangements

Billing as Work Progresses—Generally a patient is billed once a month.

Two or Three Payment Plan—Payments spaced according to agreement by patient and office dental auxiliary.

Extended Payment Plan—From three to ten payments spaced according to agreement.

Payment by Bank Loan—The doctor may make arrangements with the bank to cover the loan made to the patient.

Payments by Third Party:

Insurance Plans Covering Dental Work in Full.

Co-Insurance Plans—Requiring patients to pay part of the cost of treatment.

Double Insurance—Coverage is by two insurance companies, because both husband and wife have dental plans.

It is up to the dental assistant or office manager to present the options the doctor has decided will be offered. He or she may not wish to present all of those listed above.

After the dentist has presented the case, he or she should turn the patient over to you, with words such as "Mrs. Smith will discuss methods of payment with you." He or she will tell you or write the time required on a treatment card for your use, and the cost of the total treatment package. (In some offices the cost will be figured out by the dental assistant.)

Make sure the patient understands the treatment plan and the options for payment. Ask if he or she has any questions, and let the patient take the time necessary to digest what has been discussed. (This will prevent future difficulties and possible misunderstandings.) Don't press the patient to make a decision if he or she seems reluctant to do so. Many people want to talk the matter over with their spouses. (If a contract is a large one, you may ask the spouse to come in, so that the work to be done and the financial arrangements are understood fully.)

After the matter is settled, fill out and have the patient sign a Truth-in-Lending form. This is necessary if any service fee is charged, if any delinquency fee is charged, if there are four or more payments, or if the amount of an installment is charged. Give the patient a copy of the form, and two appointment cards for the first two appointments.

A few "no-nos."

Don't convince a patient to accept a fee higher than he or she can afford—according to what he or she tells you.

Don't arrange for larger payments than the patient can handle.

Don't "hard sell." The public relations aspect of finances must be considered.

Don't let financial arranging embarrass or intimidate you. Be firm but friendly.

If insurance forms must be filled out, do so immediately.

Don't rely on the patient to ask about co-insurances. Question him or her—just in case. It is an excellent practice builder if a patient learns he or she can have all the necessary work covered by insurance when he or she does not expect it.

Don't try to fill out insurance forms quickly. Be extremely careful when working on them since many companies will not honor claims which are not filled out perfectly or completely.

Financial record keeping by an accountant.   An accountant is often employed by the doctor. The office manager turns over to the accountant a record of the daily financial transactions, in terms of the charges and the collections. It is the accountant who keeps the books, recording all transactions. Frequently the accountant will instruct the office manager about other information he will require at regular intervals.

The office manager writes checks to pay bills, sends out monthly statements to patients owing money, takes care of petty cash, and writes checks to pay salaries.

Forensic dentistry.   This is the legal aspect of dentistry. Often dentists are able to assist the authorities in controversial criminal cases such as homicides. They also can help in the identification of victims of fires, airplane crashes and other disasters. Forensic dentists use the victims' jawbones and teeth recovered from the site of the disaster and compare them with dental x-rays on file with the person's dentist.

Forms, typing on duplicates.   Typing on several copies of forms at one time, which is something you are called upon frequently to do, can be simplified in the following ways:

Forms

1. Check the alignment by holding several copies up to the light before typing on them. If it is more convenient to do so , hold them against a window pane.

2. If you have difficulty placing all of the forms, with carbon paper between them, into the typewriter, try this: Insert the forms, without carbons, into the feed roll. Feed the paper sheets just far enough for the feed rollers to grip them. Now turn all the pages toward you, so they are draped over the front of your typewriter. Pull the pages to the back of the typewriter one sheet at a time. Insert a carbon shiny side toward you. Do this until all of the sheets are leaning back. Then roll the entire pack to the first entry.

3. To be sure the forms are aligned correctly, you may wish to give this material the "pin test." Roll the material halfway down. Put a pin through the forms at a specific point near one of the margins, near the top of the pages. You can easily see if your duplicates are in line with the top sheet. If not, you can adjust the papers.

4. If your typewriter doesn't hold the papers tightly, more "pin tests" and adjustments may be needed.

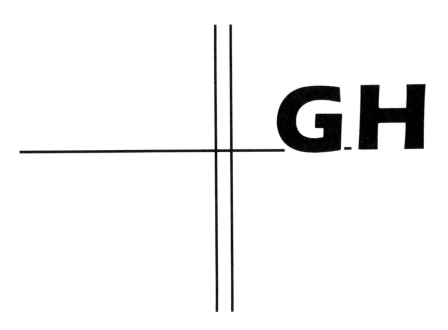

G·H

Grams to ounces conversion. To convert grams to ounces, divide by 30. To convert ounces to grams, multiply by 30.

Hepatitis B, prevention of. There is now a vaccine available (*Heptovax* B, produced by **Merck Sharp and Dohme**) which has proved to be 96 percent effective in preventing Hepatitis B, the fourth most frequently reported infectious disease in the United States. This disease poses special risks to female dental assistants—especially those in their child-bearing years.

According to Christopher M. Martin, M.D., writing in the *Journal of the ADAA*, "Hepatitis B—possibly the most serious occupational hazard facing dental assistants today—can now be virtually eliminated." The Hepatitis B virus is capable of inducing persistent viral infection, with the risk of cirrhosis of the liver and possibly liver cancer. It is particularly dangerous because a woman may be a carrier and there is a very great probability of her unborn child being infected. The baby itself may become a carrier, or have a possible shortened life span due to chronic liver disease and liver cancer.

Hepatitis B

The vaccine was licensed by the Federal Food and Drug Administration in 1981, and so far has been taken by 13,000 people with no adverse side effects.

Since health-care personnel are high on the list of persons facing the hepatitis risk, vaccination has been recommended.

Any person who has had hepatitis or who is a carrier can be infectious. High-risk patients, according to the Council on Dental Association, are those who are on the kidney machine for long periods of time, those who receive frequent transfusions or blood products, drug abusers, patients in institutions for the mentally retarded and male homosexuals. (In going over the medical history you can find clues to make you suspect the possibility of hepatitis, and you can then take precautions.)

It is possible to protect yourself by wearing a face mask (the surgical type), by wearing disposable surgical gloves, and by the extremely careful sterilization of all instruments and equipment.

The sterilization may be done by boiling water for 30 minutes, by steam sterilization (121°C for 30 minutes at 15 psi), by dry heat sterilization (160°C for one hour) or by chemical vapor sterilization (132°C at 20 psi for 20 minutes).

"Sterilizing solutions" which are used at room temperatures are not true sterilizing agents, according to the ADA. These include alcohol and ammonium compounds. Disease can be transmitted even after their use because certain viruses, bacteria and spores are not killed by this type of sterilization.

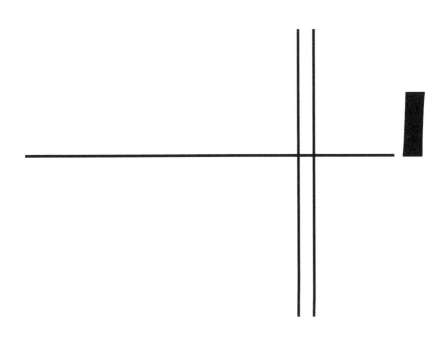

Inclement weather   During inclement weather you can save yourself time and effort by following simple procedures:

> Use a heavy pile floor mat outside the office door, so that patients and visitors can wipe their feet before entering your waiting room.

> Place an umbrella stand near the entry door, so that wet umbrellas are not carried around the room.

> Have a place close to the door where coats and hats may be put away.

> Be very much aware of wet floors (other than carpeting) because of the danger of patients' slipping. It is extremely important in winter to avoid the use of floor wax that becomes slippery when wet.

In the event that snow is predicted, and it may be necessary to close the office the next day, it is good procedure for the office manager or assistant to take home the appointment book, with patient's telephone numbers. In that case they can be called if it is not possible for the doctor to see them. This is far more preferable than if patients arrive at the office and find it closed.

Income tax deductions.   Dental auxiliaries or office managers may claim certain deductions from their income taxes. They are as follows:

> If uniforms are not provided, or paid for, their cost may be deducted. The cost of laundering them is deductible as well.
>
> The cost of any courses taken that improve one's skills for your present job are deductible. For example, if you want to take a course in filling out insurance forms, or in more efficient scheduling of patients, the Internal Revenue Service (IRS) would permit the deduction. However, the cost of courses that would prepare you for a new career are not deductible. Therefore if you were studying to become a dental laboratory technician, you could not claim those courses as deductions.
>
> Books which will be of help to you in your job may be deducted—if you purchase them.
>
> If you use your car to conduct office business (but not for going to and from work), you may deduct 16 cents per mile.
>
> The cost of supplies of any type that you purchase, and that do not come out of office funds, are deductible.

It is a good idea to speak to the person who prepares your income tax returns for other possible deductions or advice.

Income tax deductions for dental auxiliaries.   Most common deductions taken by dental auxiliaries:

> 1. fees to employment agencies and other costs incurred in order to get a new job in your present trade or profession
> 2. educational expenses such as tuition, books, laboratory fees and other expenses for courses taken which give you skills for your present trade or profession
> 3. dues to professional organizations (ADAA, for example)
> 4. uniforms and shoes and related apparel
> 5. subscriptions to professional journals
> 6. books purchased to expand your knowledge in your present field
> 7. expenses incurred while attending a business or professional convocation if by so doing you will benefit or advance in your field

8. malpractice insurance
9. income tax preparation
10. child- and dependent-care costs are partially deductible.

In 1982 the current-rate employment-related expenses for the care of your child or dependent was increased from 20 to 30 percent. Since this percentage changes from time to time, check it before making out your taxes.

Increasing efficiency. The most important item we can include in this area of increasing efficiency is that you establish your priorities for each day, list them on paper and then take care of them as soon as you can. One task may take more time than another, but if you do them in order, you will accomplish what you, yourself, have decided is most important to get done.

In this way, it is the most important things that are done first. At the end of each day make a list of your priorities for the following day. Decide before leaving what must get done, and in what order. Write these things on a large sheet of paper, so that you do not have to think about them all evening. The next day you have this work sheet to refer to.

If some tasks are urgent, label them that way on your list. These tasks may include making a certain phone call, obtaining supplies or whatever. These, naturally, will be taken care of first. Next list those of second-greatest importance. Finally list those you should get done if it is at all possible.

The next morning review the list and make any additions necessary. Check with your doctor to find out if there are tasks he or she requires you to do—and which category they fit into.

If you find you cannot finish all your work, over a period of time, you can use your work sheets to prove to your employer that you are in need of help, and you can suggest employing a part-timer.

Individualizing attention. Patients react extremely well to individualized attention. Here are some ways in which to do this:

First, listen very carefully to the patient's dental history; this will give you much information. Is this person frightened?

Has he or she gone from one dentist to another? Is his or her threshold of pain very low? Is his or her dental-hygiene routine adequate? The replies to these questions will help you to get a picture of the patient which can then be utilized when the dentist is formulating his or her treatment plan.

Next, after the plan has been made, it should be fully explained to the patient. This includes mentioning the times he or she may feel discomfort. A signal such as raising the hand may be used to give the patient a feeling of control over the situation.

After each treatment the patient should be asked, "How are you feeling now?" In this way the feedback received may be used to prescribe medication for the patient if necessary, or to reinforce the concept that you are really concerned about his or her welfare.

It is concern for the individual which is of great importance today. Most dental assistants feel it, but some, because of the daily pressures, fail to show it.

Individual Retirement Account (IRA). If you are employed, you are eligible to open an Individual Retirement Account. This is a method for preparing for your future, and, at the same time, saving on income taxes.

This is how an IRA works: You open an IRA account. You are able to place up to a maximum of $2,000 ($2,500 if spouse is unemployed) per year in that account. You are able to invest this money in a great many ways, so that it will earn the maximum amount of interest during the years it will be invested. We suggest you investigate as many sources as possible. (Many are advertised in the large-circulation newspapers, such as *The New York Times,* Sunday edition).

Banks, or money market accounts, for example, are possibilities. You pay no income tax on either the money invested or the income it earns provided you do not touch it until retirement.

You are then able to deduct the $2,000 from your taxable income. It is assumed you will be in a lower tax bracket when you retire, and therefore will pay less tax on this money that you have put away. (If you are married, you and your husband may deposit $4,000 in an IRA.)

Remember, this money must remain on deposit until you are 60 years of age. If you are forced to withdraw it, you must pay income tax on it. In addition to that you may lose money because there are penalties for early withdrawal of funds. It is, therefore, advisable to set up your IRA only if you feel you will be able to leave the money on deposit until you reach retirement age.

You can open an IRA any time up until April 15 for the previous year. This is an advantage since the fiscal year ends by December 31. You have the additional three and one-half months to set aside the money required and get the account started.

Installment payment. It may be advisable for your doctor to establish a system of installment payments. Certainly a cash practice is to be desired, but it may be impossible to maintain, particularly during a period of inflation or recession.

Determine, with the doctor, in advance, what the first payment must be (in terms of a percentage of the entire bill) and then what subsequent payments (also percentage wise) should be. There are some dentists who require the entire bill be paid in advance, or the entire laboratory fee, or a certain percentage of the fee.

Your employer may decide to utilize a credit card system. This has been a help to patients accustomed to this type of credit. Other dentists suggest patients take out bank loans, and find this effective. In this case the bank loans the money, but it is guaranteed by the doctor; (of course the patient is unaware of this guarantee.) In this way a patient who might be considered by the bank to be a bad risk is still able to borrow money to pay his bill.

Payments should not be spread over a period longer than a year. That should be your absolute maximum and even that should not be encouraged.

It is, however, worthwhile to present financial alternatives. Professionals have found that patients may be encouraged to pay their bills in full by offering a five percent discount. You can explain this by saying, "We can offer this discount because our bookkeeping is simplified and time is saved when bills are paid promptly."

Instructions to patient. It is your responsibility to give patients their instructions for postoperative care. The most effective way in which this should be done is to take a two-fold approach.

Instructions should be given in writing. Possibly you may have these printed up in advance. If not, they should be written carefully and legibly. If a prescription for medication is given it should be written by you and signed by the doctor. This is a great timesaver.

In addition to these written instructions, verbal instructions should also be given. This involves your talking through exactly what is written on the paper. Invite the patient to ask questions, and, if you aren't sure the patient understands exactly what he or she must do, then question him or her. Review each item or procedure involved in the instructions.

By following this procedure you can help the patient to avoid errors, and you can possibly help him or her to avoid pain or discomfort. Furthermore, it is entirely possible that you'll eliminate the need for the patient to telephone frantically with an emergency in the middle of the night.

Instruments, dental. Our discussion of the most frequently used dental instruments will be grouped by the procedures in which they are used. (In the illustrations which follow, some instruments are shown without the long handles they usually have to show detail.)

Examination:

Explorer—the instrument used to probe the enamel crown of the tooth to detect caries.

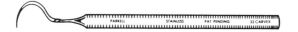

86

Mouth mirror—used for vision and for the protection and retraction of the soft tissues.

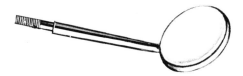

Periodontal probe (often referred to as simply "probe")—used to chart the depth of the periodontal pocket and abnormalities of the gums. These may be calibrated with engraved lines or bands of color.

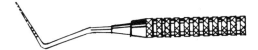

Cotton pliers (often referred to as "college pliers")—used to transfer medication, absorbent cotton or gutta percha points, and cotton pellets to the operating field. These instruments may have a lock on the handle.

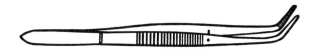

Operative dentistry:

Spoon excavator—used to remove decayed tooth structure from the cavity preparation.

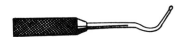

Instruments, dental

Amalgam carrier—used to transfer amalgam to the cavity preparation. This instrument is available in different sizes, in single and double ends and is made of plastic or metal. The carrier is loaded by pressing the tip into the amalgam mix with the lever on the stem locked open with your thumb.

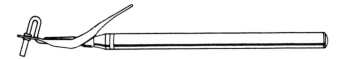

Amalgam plugger—used to pack the amalgam into the preparation.

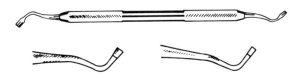

Amalgam carver—used to remove excess amalgam after the cavity is filled. The type of blade used is a matter of the dentist's preference.

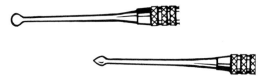

Burnisher—used to smooth superficially polished silver restoration.

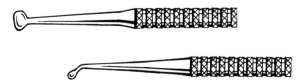

Plastic instrument—used to manipulate composite filling materials.

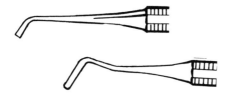

Hatchets and Hoes—Used to finish the preparation by removing unsupported enamel and adding angulation to the floor of the proximal preparation.

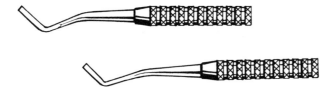

Periodontics:

Currette—used to do root planing and to remove subgingival calculus; the currette also, because of its blade angulation, removes the diseased soft tissue of the pocket.

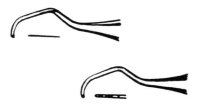

Chisel—used to remove large calculus deposits by breaking them up. Chisels are used for deposits in the anterior section of the mouth.

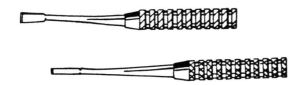

Instruments, dental

Scalers—used to remove supragingival calculus. The blades are varied to provide access to all surfaces of the teeth.

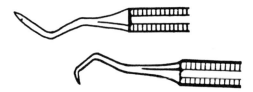

Periosteal elevator—used to retract and protect the gingiva after it has been incised to provide access to the root surface and alveolar bone.

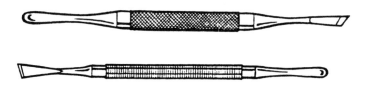

Knives—used to incise tissue that will then be discarded. They come in various shapes to accomodate access to various areas of the mouth.

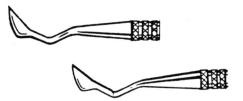

Scalpels—used to incise the soft tissue when performing surgery. These are often disposable.

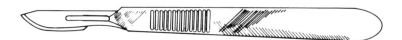

Rongeur forceps—used to remove bone. The blade of these forceps cuts when they are closed. This instrument is also used after extraction to remove or reshape the alveolar crest.

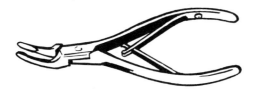

Endodontics:

Explorer—used to probe for the entrance (orifice) of the root canal after excavating the tooth. Explorers are often double-ended instruments.

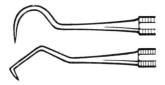

Irrigating Syringe—used to carry medicaments or solutions to the root canal.

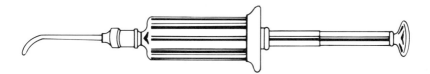

Endodontic hand instruments—used to remove the pulp and smooth the walls of the root canal. All are thin pieces of wire embedded in colored plastic handles. Canals are instrumented in a sequence of increasing diametered instruments; the colored plastic handles are coded. The colors used are purple, white, yellow, red, blue, green, black, as the diameter of the instrument increases in size. The purple-handled

91

instrument begins at .05mm. at the tip and increases to .35mm. The white-handled instrument ranges for .40mm up. The length of these instruments is the other criterion that is used to differentiate them. They are usually available in 21 and 25 mm. lengths, with longer instruments available as special sets, which are rarely needed.

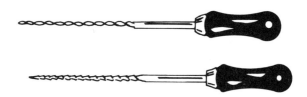

Endodontic k-file—used by being inserted in the canal, which is then x-rayed to determine the location of the apex of the tooth. These have very little cutting capacity.

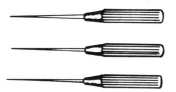

Endodontic broach—this barbed instrument is used to engage and remove the dental pulp from the canal.

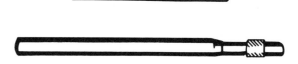

Hedstrom files—used to cut and remove the rough dentin from the canal.

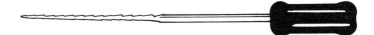

Spreader—used to spread the gutta percha point to assure even filling of the canal.

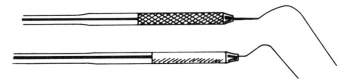

Rubber dam—many practitioners perform all intracanal procedures with the rubber dam. Please check the separate entry for details of placement and instrumentation needed.

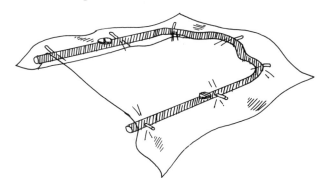

Oral surgery:

Elevators—used to aid in extractions by being placed between the tooth and the alveolus and loosening the tooth prior to placing the forceps. There are a variety of types of elevators available for various purposes. Often when the tip of the root is broken during an extraction, elevators are used to remove the fragments.

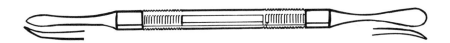

Extraction forceps—used to remove the tooth. There are many different types of forceps available for both the deciduous and permanent dentition. In general, the more extractions your employer performs, the fewer forceps he will regularly use, both for simplicity and economy. You should find out which types are kept in the office, and list them by number and function. Post this list where it is available for you to consult when necessary.

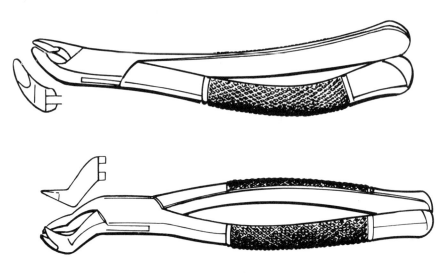

Instrument passing. The assistant who is alert and responsible to her chair-side duties is always thinking one step ahead of the dentist. Working as a team on procedures that are being constantly repeated, it will not be long before you can virtually anticipate every request and have the instrument or material ready at hand before being asked.

Instruments should be transferred with one hand. The assistant should position her hand below the patient's chin, with the fingers pointing at the doctor. Instruments are transferred with the working end toward the patient so the dentist can use them right away.

Instrument set-ups. One of the most important tasks you, as a dental assistant, will be called upon to do is set up trays of instruments for the doctor to use. Since different instruments and materials are needed for the various procedures, it is necessary to be very specific in preparing these set-ups.

You will find listed below the instruments the doctor will probably need in order to do specific types of work. Check to be sure you include everything required by reviewing this listing with him or her.

Then post the listing in the sterilization area, so that it may be referred to whenever necessary. It is particularly valuable when personnel are new, and not fully trained. Nothing is more annoying than a situation in which the doctor does not have the items needed when he or she is working on a patient.

Amalgams

Mirror	Explorer	Saliva ejector
Cotton pliers	Condensors	Carrier
Cotton rolls	Carbide burs	Tofflemire or other
Matrix bands	Wedges	matrix retainer
Articulating paper	Burnishers	Squeeze cloth
Cavity liner or base	Cavity varnish	Amalgam carrier

Composite fillings

Mirror	Explorer	Burs No. _____
Cotton pliers	Rubber dam	Mixing instruments
Composite paste and liquids	Shade guide	Plastic instruments
Slab	Spatula	Cellophane strips
Light curing source	Saliva ejector	Polishing strips

Inlays

Mirror	Explorer	Burs No. _____
Cotton pliers	Cotton rolls	Temporary filling material
Diamond stones No. _____	Wax	Gingival packing string
Chisels	Local anesthetic	
	Trimmers	
Impression materials	Saliva ejector	Impression trays

Instrument set-ups

Porcelain Jacket or Individual Crown Preparation

Mirror	Explorer	Bite-recording
Burs No. _____	Diamond stones	material
Impression materials	No. _____	Saliva ejector
Gingival packing	Impression trays	Local anesthetic
string	Self-curing acrylic	Temporary cement
Shade guide	Articulating paper	Crown forms
Paper pad		Wax

Crown and Bridge (Preparation)

Mirror	Bite-recording	Cement pads
Local anesthetic	materials	Saliva ejector
Diamond stones	Explorer	Burs No. _____
No. _____	Cotton pliers	Shade guide
Impression materials	Wax	Impression loading
Temporary bridge	Impression trays	syringes
materials	Gingival packing	Articulating paper
	string	

Crown and Bridge (Cementation)

Mirror	Slab or pad	Wooden bite stick
Cotton pliers	Crown remover	Stones
Explorer	Polishing agent	Cement spatula
Cotton rolls	Diamond stones	Cement liquid
Saliva ejector	No. _____	Articulating paper
Cement instrument	Cement powder	

Full Denture (Primary Impression)

Impression trays	Compound	Alcohol lamp and
Wax spatula	Wax	torch
Water heater	Compound heater	

Full Denture (Secondary Impression)

Mirror

Customized or stock impression tray

Wax spatula

Mixing instruments

Explorer

Impression paste

Alcohol lamp and torch

Cotton pliers

Beading wax

Mixing pad

Full Denture (Vertical and Centric)

Mirror

Bite rims

Alcohol torch

Millimeter ruler

Tooth mold

Explorer

Base plate wax

Indelible pencil

Wax spatula

Shade guides

Cotton pliers

Face bow

Caliper

Wax carver

Full Denture (Try-In)

Mirror

Wax spatula

Hand mirror

Explorer

Wax

Denture adhesive

Cotton pliers

Bunsen burner

Full Denture (Insertion)

Mirror

Heatless and carborundum stones

Pressure-indicator paste

Explorer

Articulating paper

Hand mirror

Cotton pliers

Pumice

Diamond stones

Full Denture (Adjustment)

Mirror

C C trimmers

Carborundum stones

Explorer

Articulating paper

Indelible pencil

Cotton pliers

Heatless stones

Pressure-indicator paste

Instrument set-ups

Partial Denture (Impressions)

Mirror	Explorer	Cotton pliers
Alginate (premeasured)	Perforated trays	Rubber bowl
Spatula	Room-temperature water	

Partial Denture (Vertical and Centric)

Mirror	Explorer	Cotton pliers
Wax rims	Wax	Wax spatula
Matches	Bunsen burner	Alcohol torch

Partial Denture (Try-In)

Mirror	Explorer	Wax spatula
Wax	Bunsen burner	Matches
Articulating paper		

Partial Denture (Insertion)

Mirror	Explorer	Cotton pliers
Heatless stones	Carborundum stones	Articulating paper
Mouth rinse	Hand mirror	

Periodontal Surgery

Mirror	Explorer	Scaling instruments
Pocket probes	Gingival pack	Mixing pad
Gingival knives	Diamond bone burs	Suture needle
Blades No. _____	No. _____	Scissors
Suture thread No. _____	Needle holder	
	Cotton pliers	

Extractions

Mirror	Explorer	Saliva ejector
Cotton pliers	Sterile sponges	Gelfoam
Elevators No. _____	(2 x 2″)	Bone file
Curettes	Forceps	

Prophylaxis

Mirror	Explorer	Cotton pliers
Scalers No. _____	Pumice	Prophylaxis angle
Rubber clips	Porte polisher	Plastic drape
Ultrasonic sealer	Ultrasonic tips No. _____	

Root Canal

Rubber Dam	Rubber dam clamps	Burs No. _____
Broaches No. _____	Reamers No. _____	Files No. _____
Cement instruments	Paper points	Medicaments
Cement liquid	Cement powder	Slab
Spatula	Temporary stopping	

Insulin Shock or Diabetic Coma.   Diabetics are subject to insulin shock if too much insulin or too little food is taken. It is characterized by weakness, moist skin, and a full, bounding pulse. These patients require immediate administration of sugar or glucose. Orange juice is often given under these circumstances.

Diabetic patients suffering from elevated blood sugar caused by inadequate insulin in the body may be confused, suffer from nausea or vomiting, feel ill, have dry mouth and skin and be extremely thirsty. Their blood pressure may be low and their pulse weak and rapid.

In these cases, the doctor or an ambulance should be summoned immediately.

If a patient is known to be diabetic and appears to be in

trouble, it is best to administer orange juice and sugar immediately, because high blood sugar is less dangerous than low blood sugar.

A diabetic in a state of coma is a medical emergency necessitating immediate hospitalization.

Check these instructions with your employer.

Insurance. The filling out of insurance forms has become one of the major tasks of the office manager. It is essential that you understand the forms and mechanisms used to file these forms, and how to obtain maximum benefits for the patient.

You must first realize that dental coverage varies arbitrarily from insurance company to insurance company. Accordingly, one mechanism you may use when filing a claim is to presubmit an estimate of services and their cost for prior approval by the insurance company. Since the maximum payment a company will tender is often less than the doctor's fee for the service, and the patient will be expected to make up the difference, precertifying claims will allow you to inform the patient of this and arrange payment of the balance while treatment progresses. While this is especially important in expensive cases where considerable work is to be done, it is also valuable when you are unfamiliar with a given company's policies. Recently, a patient the author had fabricated partial dentures for had his claim disallowed. The company refused payment because the dentist had not extracted any teeth prior to inserting the dentures. If experience tells you that there is any question as to a company paying benefits, have the estimate submitted first.

There are basically two ways in which benefits are dispersed—the patient may be paid directly, or the check sent to the office. Payment directly to the dentist, which is preferable, involves having the patient sign a statement to the effect on the form submitted to the company. Using this method reduces any time and effort spent in collecting; patients have been known to hold back the check after receiving it.

The insurance form itself, while differing in format from company to company, usually has a section that must be completed by the patient, which includes basic data such as his or her employer, their address, age and other background. The section you will fill out will usually involve a dental chart and space to list procedures that are to be done. Use the master file to fill in this section. Also, you will find a space for the ADA code numbers for each procedure. These are a chart of common dental procedures that the American Dental Association has developed to facilitate and standardize for the insurance companies. Often, the code is printed on the back of the insurance form; if not, be sure you have a copy of these codes at hand.

You may be directed, or choose to submit, study models and x-rays. Models should always be well packed and insulated so that no part of either model is touching, which prevents breakage in the mail. X-rays should be mailed with a note on the envelope—"X-rays — do not bend."

In time you will develop a good idea of the character of each different company. As a precaution against "loss" of the claim, we recommend you photocopy the completed form and leave a copy with the patient's chart, just in case.

Finally, it should be noted that since third-party payment (that is, payment by an insurance company) has become very popular within the last twenty years, there is an art to learning how to fill out the forms to insure the patient receives the most he or she is entitled to. Continuing-education courses in this subject are available, and we feel any money spent on this by your employer is a good investment, and we heartily endorse this.

Insurance book.   Often simple devices can be of great help. Such a device is the insurance book.

Use a notebook for this purpose. Devote a page to each day. On that page indicate the name of every patient seen that day who has dental insurance. Also put in the name of the company, the date the claim was filed and to whom benefits are assigned. If co-insurance is available, that should be indicated as well.

Because this information is in one place, the need to pull out files is eliminated.

When bills are sent out, check the book to learn how much time has elapsed since the form was sent in, and to see that if you must take further action you are made aware of it.

Any dealings you have regarding the particular patient and the insurance company should be indicated in the notebook.

Insurance plans. Many patients have little or no idea to which benefits they are entitled. It is well worth your time and effort to explain exactly and specifically what their coverage entitles them to.

When a patient comes into the office, you can ask if he or she has insurance coverage. Find out what it is, and explain as much as you can about it. In this way you can avoid problems later on, such as the patient suddenly learning he or she is not covered for a particular situation.

If possible, determine which dental insurance plans are to be found in your community, and learn as much as you can about them.

Your local chapter of the **American Dental Association** can prove to be very helpful in this regard. Contact them for assistance.

Integrity in filling out forms. There is rarely a dentist who has not been asked to request payment from an insurance company by a patient for services not rendered to that particular person. It may be for services rendered to a member of that person's family, but, unless the policy specifically covers the situation, you cannot do this.

Many people do not realize at what point benefits to their children are no longer paid. They, too, expect you to request benefits.

Your response, when requests of either type mentioned above are made, should be, "I'm very sorry, but we cannot possibly do this for any of our patients because it is illegal. We simply cannot make any statements which are not true."

Do not allow any patient to talk you into doing this, because your employer could be prosecuted for this.

This is not to say that you do not try to obtain as much coverage for the patient as he or she is entitled to. This is a service to which the patient is entitled, but it must be completely legal and above board.

Inventory. The following is a listing of supplies commonly used in most dental offices. Check with your doctor to determine which are to be omitted, and which others are to be added.

This inventory of supplies may be used in one of two ways. You may type up a list, and then check off those supplies you have on hand, or you may indicate those which are missing.

It is a good idea to use several carbons—so that you do not have to type the list more often than three times a year. You may also type one list, and then have twelve columns, one for each month, or make photocopies for a year in advance.

Office supplies:

Letterheads _____

Envelopes
    Small _____
    Large _____
    Glass enclosures _____

Memo pads

Patient record cards

Appointment cards

Scotch tape

Paper clips
    Large _____
    Small _____

Typewriter ribbons or
    cartridges _____

Pens _____

Pencils _____

Postage Stamps _____

Banking supplies
    Checks _____
    Deposit slips _____

Basic supplies:

Tissues _____

Paper towels _____

Toilet paper _____

Garbage bags _____

Liquid soap _____

Rubber gloves _____

Glove powder _____

Surgical drapes _____

Sutures _____

Treatment supplies:

Gauze, 2 x 2's _____

Amalgam _____

Composite _____

Vaseline gauze _____

103

Inventory

Treatment supplies (continued):

Cotton-tip applicators _____   Impression materials _____

Tape _____   Blades _____

Tongue blades _____   Alcohol _____

Cotton balls _____   Spirits of ammonia _____

Cotton rolls _____   Vaseline (Sterile) _____

Syringes _____   Root Canal supplies _____

Crowns and crown   Formalin _____

  forms _____   Acetic acid _____

Burs _____   Needles _____

Medicines and Injectables:

Anesthetics _____   Atropine _____

Gentian violet _____   Scopolamine _____

Penicillin _____   Ethyl chloride _____

Erythromycin _____   ASA compound _____

Tetracycline _____   Empirin compound _____

Topical Anesthetics _____   Empirin compound with

Local Anesthetics _____   codeine _____

Phenobarbitol _____   Lincomycin _____

Seconal _____   Tylenol with codeine _____

104

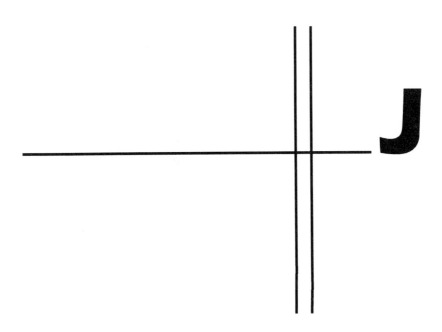

Job applicants, advertising for. Placing an advertisement, the following points should be included:

1. Nature of the job: (e.g., Dental assistant, Dental receptionist, Dental office manager, or Dental hygienist).

2. Experienced or nonexperienced?

3. A description of the hours of employment (e.g., Full time 9-5, half day Saturday).

4. A brief description of the skills required (e.g., If experience is essential, it should be stated).

5. Any special requirements. (e.g., Must relate well to senior citizens.)

6. Your employer may wish to state the salary, but this is not necessary. It is customary to do so in some sections of the country, and rarely so in others.

7. Ask for a resumé, and a telephone number.

8. Give a box number to which applicants are to write. (Unless it is essential the job be filled quickly, this is far preferable to giving a telephone number.)

Work up the advertisement before placing it, and have your employer check the copy and approve it.

Job applicants—application

Keep a copy of the advertisement in your file, so that it may be reused when necessary.

When screening replies, first read through the replies and separate those in which you are interested from those in which you are not. Then review the letters and resumés carefully. Check for the points listed below, and group the responses into first and second choice.

> The type of experience or background that fits your office's needs
>
> Correct spelling and punctuation
>
> The cleanliness and neatness of the reply
>
> Proper use of language

Do not discard any letters, however, until a final selection is made since it may be necessary to return to the second group at some point.

Telephone the possible employees. Ask them several questions to get some idea of their speech. If it is acceptable, ask them to come in for a *preliminary interview*. Make sure this is understood, thereby avoiding any possibility of a misunderstanding.

Job applicants—application. Prepare an application that should be duplicated and used whenever anyone applies for a position.

There are certain points of information which, according to law, may not be asked. These have been avoided in the form that follows:

1. Name.
2. Marital state: Check one.
   Married _____, Separated, divorced or widowed _____, Single _____
3. Have you any children? If so, state their names and ages.
4. Education: Check the appropriate space.
   High school graduate _____
   Two years or less or college _____
   Three years or less of college _____
   College graduate: School _____

106

Year _____
Special training: School _____
Year _____

5. Employment. List all previous positions, including years worked and reason for leaving.

6. Interests and hobbies.

7. References. List three people who may be contacted, who are not relatives, and who have known you at least five years. Give their mailing addresses and telephone numbers.

After the preliminary interview prepare for each applicant a "package" to give to the doctor, consisting of the original letter, the resumé and your evaluation sheet.

It should be the doctor's job to hire personnel, not that of the office manager or assistant—unless otherwise decided upon.

As soon as reference replies come in, give them to the doctor. No one should be hired permanently until all references are in and have been checked.

Job applicant—interviewing. As office manager, it may be necessary for you to screen a number of job applicants. To do so efficiently, give each a specific appointment. Since this is the preliminary interview, 30 minutes should be more than enough time. Have the applicant fill out the application form (see listing).

It will save time if you give a type-written description of the job to each applicant. Discuss the type of practice and the requirements for fulfilling the job.

Encourage the applicant to ask questions, and to discuss his or her background. Get applicants to talk, so that you can evaluate their ability to communicate.

You may wish to prepare a checklist which will enable you to very quickly evaluate every applicant after you have talked with him or her. The following points should be included:

1. Punctuality: on time___ ten minutes late ___ more than ten minutes late ___

2. Appearance: excellent ___ good ___ acceptable ___ unacceptable ___

3. Ability to communicate: excellent ___ good ___ acceptable ___ unacceptable ___

4. Personality: excellent ___ good ___ acceptable ___ unacceptable ___

5. Experience: excellent ___ good ___ acceptable ___ unacceptable ___

6. Skills: _____

7. Speed of movement: excellent ___ good ___ acceptable ___ unacceptable ___

8. Interest in job: excellent ___ good ___ acceptable ___ unacceptable ___

9. Possible problems:
   (e.g. Young children—who will care for them?)
   (Overweight—careless personal habits.)

10. General impression:

This checklist is only for your eyes and for your employer's. Be absolutely certain that no one else ever sees it! Remember you may be working with this person in the future.

The checklist may be destroyed after a person is hired. If you wish it kept, place it where it is safe from prying eyes.

After the interviews, tell the applicants approximately when they will be contacted. Thank them for coming in, and tell them you enjoyed meeting them. Leave them with a favorable impression of you and the office, regardless of whether they are being considered for the job.

For those applicants whom you are seriously considering, a check of all references is essential. It is best for your communication to be in writing, with a written reply requested.

You may use a letter (on office letterhead) such as the following. Enclose a stamped self-addressed envelope, as well. This will do much toward your receiving a reply.

Dear _____ :

_____ has applied for a position on our staff and has given your name as a reference. May we ask you to complete the following and return to us in the enclosed, stamped envelope. As you know, we must depend on your assistance and thank you for it.

Please rate the person named above by checking one of the following. Should you care to add comments, do not hesitate to do so.

1. Appearance—on a daily basis:
   excellent __ good __ fair __ poor __
2. Ability to relate to the public:
   excellent __ good __ fair __ poor __
3. Ability to work with others on staff:
   excellent __ good __ fair __ poor __
4. Punctuality:
   excellent __ good __ fair __ poor __
5. Cleanliness
6. Interest in job
7. Intelligence—use of it
8. Absence record

Above all, we must know if you consider this applicant honest and trustworthy. Yes __ No __

Any visible problems?
Additional comments (Typist—leave space)

Our sincere thanks for your cooperation.

Very truly yours,
Dr. XYZ

(Have the doctor sign these letters, or authorize you to sign his name.)

If a person is being seriously considered, the doctor may wish to telephone her previous employer. Often, information a former employer may be reluctant to put into writing will be given verbally to the doctor.

Job applicants, sources.

1. You may have, among the doctor's patients, persons whom you feel would be an asset to your staff. It is certainly worthwhile to approach them, asking if they are interested. If so, they should be given an application form (see listing).

2. You may consult the "position's wanted" listing of newspapers for possible candidates.

3. You may consult employees of other offices for leads. (Be careful, however, that you are not accused of "head hunting" or stealing employees from other dentists.)

4. You may have friends or acquaintances whom you feel would be worthwhile candidates. You may invite them to apply for the position, but it is advisable to make sure they realize you cannot guarantee they will be hired.

5. Your employer may prefer to work with an employment agency.

6. Your employer may wish to have an advertisement placed in your local newspaper, or other publications (see listing).

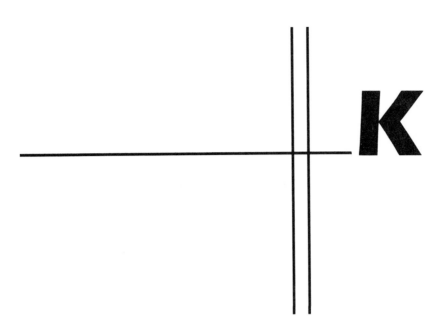

Keeping patient records. Whenever an addition is made to a patient's record, it should be dated and information such as the following should be added: All reports of laboratory tests, X-ray findings, and reports of other doctors.

After each office visit, a notation should be made of the date and the condition of the patient, indicating the progress of the case and the procedures performed by the dentist that day. Again question the patient regarding drug allergies or changes in the medical history.

Make note of telephone calls as well as office visits. Label the former with letters (T.C.). Do not fail to do this. It is important.

Periodically check the patient's address and telephone number.

If a patient fails to keep an appointment, or fails to follow through on the doctor's orders, note this on his or her record. This information can be of great help if the doctor continues to treat the patient.

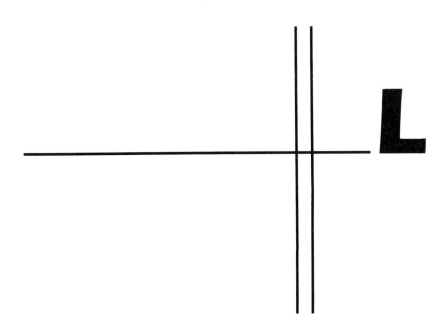

Labeled items. All medications and other materials you use must be labeled clearly. A number of toxic materials are clear, colorless, odorless liquids. To keep the original label as clean and legible as possible, cover it with transparent cellophane tape. When pouring the contents from the bottle, hold your hand on the label and pour down the opposite side.

If a label is missing or is not legible, discard the material in the container. Do not take any chances on remembering the contents.

If a label is messy, type up another, copying all of the information from the original onto the new one.

If you use a large supply bottle and small, handy bottles for everyday use, be careful that the labeling is easy to read and the correct materials are poured from one container to the other.

Latecomers, working with. As office manager, you sometimes deal with patients who are late for their appointments, and no one knows better than you how upsetting this is. There are several steps you can take to remedy this.

First talk to the patient. Point out his or her needs. Explain that these dental appointments are really important because their mouth and teeth are seriously in need of the care being given them. If you are able to impress the patient with the *importance* of treatment, you may be able to change his or her habits.

If speaking to this type of patient doesn't help, schedule them for a specific time, but tell them a half hour earlier (or an hour—depending on how late they usually arrive). For instance, Jim Brown is frequently an hour late. Schedule him for 2 P.M. but tell him 1 P.M. Don't let him get any indication that you are doing this! Indicate 2 P.M. in your appointment book. For example, place the letter E 1 P.M. next to the 2 P.M. The E means you've told Jim "earlier," at 1 P.M. Then, should he telephone, you will know at a glance what the situation is. Do not be afraid to do this. It works well with some late-comers. There is also no serious problem if the patient must wait for the doctor. That is preferable to having the doctor's schedule disrupted.

Letters, forms of.   There are several styles from which you may choose for your correspondence:

1. *Full-block style:* Every part of the letter, including date, name, and address of the recipient, salutation, message, the complimentary closing and signature begins at the left margin.

2. *Block style:* This form is similar to the full-block style except that the date and the complimentary close and signature are placed three inches from the right margin. The remaining parts of the letter start at the left margin.

3. *Nonblock style:* In this form the date, the complimentary close and the signature are placed three inches from the right margin.
   The name and address of the recipient and the salutation are at the left margin. The first sentence of each paragraph is indented. After that all of the material begins at the left margin.

Any of these forms is correct, and you may use whichever you prefer. See sample letters, p.115.

Full block style

January 2, 19

Dr. John Smith
234 Main Street
New York, NY 10053

Dear Dr. Smith,
Thank you very much for referring Mary Jones to us for treatment.
We will do everything we can to justify your confidence in us.

Sincerely yours,
Frank Brown, D.D.S.

Block style

January 2, 19

Dr. John Smith
234 Main Street
New York, NY 10053;

Dear Dr. Smith,
Thank you very much for referring Mary Jones to us for treatment.
We will do everything we can to justify your confidence in us.

Sincerely yours,
Frank Brown, D.D.S.

Nonblock style

January 2, 19

Dr. John Smith
234 Main Street
New York, NY 10053

Dear Dr. Smith,
   Thank you very much for referring Mary Jones to us for treatment. We will do everything we can to justify your confidence in us.

Very truly yours,
Frank Brown, D.D.S.

Letter writing.   There are several forms of business letters, as shown on page 115, which are acceptable. You may find the Full-Block Style, straight line, newer form enables you to save time. (See Letters, forms of.)

Use forms whenever possible.   Develop forms which you can reuse over and over again. This can be done by keeping previously written letters on hand, and making the appropriate changes. You will find sample forms in this book under the following entries: Collections letter, appointment letter, thank you for referrals letter.

Keep your language clear and simple. Your prime purpose in writing is to communicate well, and to get specific ideas across to the person reading your letter.

In sending out office mail, use stationery with an office letterhead. Advise your doctor to have printed 6 x 9" as well as 8½ x 11" stationery. Never use any scrap or cheap paper for sending notes out of the office. Your letters represent your employer, and should do so in the best possible light.

Make sure your typewriter is clean, and the ribbon inked. A faint impression is difficult to read, *and* poor public relations.

Proofread every piece of typed or written material you send out. When dates are included, check these carefully. Make sure your spelling is correct.

Linens.   Many doctors have services which supply their linens. Each week soiled linen is picked up, and fresh linen is delivered. This service should be checked to see that the correct number of items is delivered, and that the linen is not torn or stained.

If your doctor does not use a service, but uses a laundry instead, you will have to list the items you send. Then, when the laundry is returned, you must check to be sure all of it has been returned. Some laundries request a list accompany the soiled linen.

Each day put out fresh towels for the doctor and a fresh office coat, if he or she wears one.

During the day the assistant must check the condition of the towels. As soon as they are stained they should be replaced.

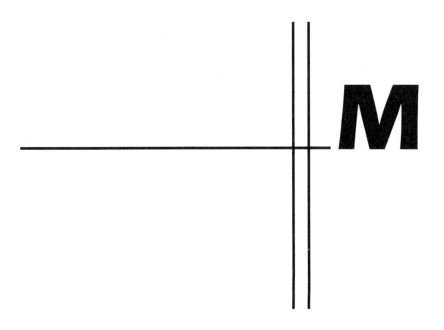

Magazines. It is the office manager's responsibility to keep the waiting room material up to date. This involves ordering subscriptions and removing out-of-date publications. Generally, magazines of various types are used, and should be kept in a rack where they are easily available.

Selection should be made depending on the clientele. If it is predominantly women, several magazines of news and home decoration, one or two revolving around people, and one or two containing fiction should be considered. For the men, sports, automobiles, or business publications are appropriate; again, the character of the patients should be taken into account.

Do not forget to include children's magazines or books. These are very important if children visit your office as patients or accompanying their parents.

Use a large rack which holds the magazines so that they are easily visible. In this way they will not appear messy, and will require less "straightening up" at the end of the day. However, if they are not neat, they should be rearranged whenever necessary. Plastic covers can help keep the magazines in good shape as well.

Discard magazines when they become tattered or torn as well as when they are outdated. A supply of interesting, current, well-cared-for publications is important.

Mail—handling incoming checks. Patient's payments in the form of checks should be entered in your Daily Account Book and on the Patient's Financial Record.

Before doing so, however, each check should be examined. This procedure takes only a minute or two, but should be done to avoid complications.

Look at the following items:

1. Date: The check should not be postdated (dated ahead). Banks do not honor postdated checks.
2. Amount: Make sure the amount of the check is the same in words as it is in numbers. (e.g. A check for $550.00/100 is not valid if the words call for "Five fifty dollars." It must read "Five hundred fifty dollars.")
3. Signature: Every check must be signed in order to be honored by a bank.
4. No check is valid if changes have been made on it—including erasures.

After this review of a check has been made it is ready to be deposited to the office account.

Mail record log. A record of all the mail the doctor receives should be kept, with entries made daily. Use a ledger with space for the date, the sender of the mail, a summary of its contents and the action taken.

Action taken may be indicated by code.

Ans = answered. Include the date of your response.
Fi = filed.
Dr. = passed along to the doctor.

The one type of mail your employer may wish to ignore is advertisements. Discuss this to determine policy.

Maintenance of patient records. It is the province of the office manager to make sure that all records are complete. Every day

118

she should check the records of each patient who was seen that day to make sure a notation was made of the date and the doctor's services rendered. At the same time she should make sure the record is in keeping with previous notations.

Remember that the patient's record is a legal document. If you have any questions, double-check with the doctor or assistant.

Manual, Procedures. Every staff member should know exactly what is expected of him or her. One way to insure this is to have a Procedures Manual, in which each person's job is spelled out in very explicit detail. In that way another person may read it and be able to perform the tasks and know his or her responsibility.

The task of developing a manual falls to the office manager. To develop a manual, begin by having each person list the tasks she performs. Index cards may be used for this. After a period of several weeks, the cards for each job should be read, and placed in the order in which the daily tasks must be done. Items which are lacking will be noticed, and may be added at any time in the future.

In the Manual, pictures of equipment are placed next to the task which utilizes them. These may be cut out of catalogs or drawn by hand.

Tasks as fundamental as turning on the lights, turning on the air conditioning and pulling up window shades should be listed.

A new person who is hired should be able to function effectively using this manual. Therefore, it should be as specific as possible regarding the tasks listed.

As dentistry is a constantly changing discipline, and as new materials and techniques are always being developed, it is wise to upgrade the manual periodically.

Matrices and retainers. When the proximal surface of a tooth needs to be filled, a retainer and matrix are used to provide a surface against which to condense the silver. This system should be prepared in advance to maximize chairside productivity.

For anterior teeth, the matrix of choice is a clear cellophane strip that is held in place with a metal clip, a wooden or plastic wedge, or the fingers. This cannot be set up in advance and is fit by the dentist in the mouth.

For posterior teeth, where the contact area is wider than in the anterior region, the matrix is metal. It is placed in a retainer and then wedged in place before the amalgam is condensed. The most common retainer used is called a Tofflemire retainer.

To prepare the retainer, first take the metal matrix and fold it in half. You will see a conical circle formed—the smaller end of the cone will always be the gingival part of the matrix. Place the doubled matrix into the slot in the body of the retainer and the conical end of the matrix through the first slot in the U-shaped end of the retainer. Then bend the matrix to the left or right, being sure to leave the slotted tip of the U empty. Then tighten the screw at the opposite end of the retainer until the matrix is locked in place. Since the matrix can only be placed to the left or right of the U slot, preparing a few of these retainers in advance covers all possible placement. The retainer is passed to the dentist, who places and then wedges it.

Matrices may be placed back to back, or on nonadjacent teeth.

Children's teeth are more bulbous at the contact area, and the doctor may choose a T-matrix for proximal fillings. This is a metal band with an overlapping T at one end. The matrix is placed by the dentist, who fits it to the tooth and bends the arms of the T over the base. In this case, simply pass the band to the dentist when he or she asks for it.

Medical history, employees. It is good prevention to have the name of the personal physician and medical history for all office employees on file should an emergency arise. If this information is not currently available, suggest it to your employer. This information can be a significant help and may prove to be important at any time. Of special importance are possible drug allergies or preexisting conditions that might appear during working hours.

Medical history, patient's. It may be part of the dental assistant's job to take a patient's medical history before he or she is seen by the dentist. The medical history is written up as the patient gives the information to you; however, in certain cases the patients may be given the form to complete by themselves. It is your responsibility to inform your employer if you have any reservations about a patient's response. Many times the patient is unsure of the correct response, or considers it an invasion of privacy to reveal certain things. You must be able to explain, translate a medical term into layperson's language and answer any question the patient may have about his or her history. Should the point arise, you may stress to the patient that all replies are strictly confidential and will never be revealed to anyone.

If your employer allows auxiliary staff to take the history, you may say, "The doctor has instructed me to ask you some questions regarding your medical history. However, should you prefer to give him (or her) the answers, that is perfectly alright."

The medical history generally contains the following topics:

Medical History

1. Reason for the visit (or this may be termed "Chief complaint"; this should be summarized in as few words as possible—for example, if the patient has a toothache—"pain from __"; or if he or she wants a cleaning—"wants prophylaxis treatment").

2. Family history relating to serious illnesses, communicable diseases and illnesses appearing in several family members. This section may appear as a list of conditions with space for a check mark for pertinent responses.

3. History of pregnancies (for women): Number of successful pregnancies, miscarriages or abortions. Be sure to include if she is now pregnant.

4. Previous illnesses: Certain illnesses can have effects many years later.

5. Previous surgery: Any surgery, however minor, should be indicated.

6. Personal habits: The use of the following should be noted with the frequency of use (monthly, weekly, daily).

Medical history, updating

Medications (indicate which)

Caffeinated drinks (which and how often)

Alcoholic beverages (indicate quantity in ounces)

Tobacco

Vitamins

7. History of allergies: This is extremely important. Ask if the patient has ever taken penicillin, and if he or she had an allergic reaction to it. Then ask about other antibiotics and drugs. Also inquire about aspirin, since a number of people cannot take it comfortably, or may not regard it as a drug. Your office may have a policy of very obviously identifying patients with allergies on the cover of the chart, using red lettering on tape or a written notation. If the patient doesn't know if he has ever taken penicillin, note this as well on the chart.

Again, if you feel that a patient is not giving you full information, make a note of this, using a code so that your doctor is aware of the situation, and may ask further questions.

Medical history, updating. It is one of the tasks of the dental assistant to question recall patients to determine if there has been any change in their medical histories. Often a patient may have been placed on medication for a condition such as high blood pressure. It is important that this be noted.

It is most important that your doctor be aware of any new medical condition which has arisen. This should be determined by asking the patient directly. "Has there been a change in your health since you were last treated here?" If the response is "Yes," follow up. It is entirely possible a heart condition may have developed, for instance.

Make sure that if changes have occurred you write them on the patient's chart, but also inform the doctor of them.

Medical specialties. It is important for all dental personnel to be familiar with the medical as well as dental specialties; they are arranged here in alphabetical order.

1. Allergist: A physician who diagnoses and treats patients who have allergies, which are hypersensitivities to such things as pollen, foods, animals, etc.

2. Anesthesiologist: A physician who administers anesthetics to render patients insensitive to pain during surgical, obstetrical and other medical procedures.

3. Dermatologist: A physician who diagnoses and treats diseases of the human skin.

4. Internist: A physician who diagnoses and treats the patient without the use of surgery.

5. Neurologist: A physician who diagnoses and treats organic diseases and disorders of the nervous system.

6. Obstetrician (Gynecologist): A physician who treats women during prenatal, natal and postnatal periods. He or she may treat patients for disease of the generative organs.

7. Opthamologist: A physician who diagnoses and treats diseases and injuries of the eye.

8. Otorhinolaryngologist: A physician who diagnoses and treats diseases of the ear, nose and throat.

9. Pathologist: A physician who studies the nature, cause and development of diseases, and structural and functional changes caused by them. He or she diagnoses from body tissue, fluids, secretions, and other specimens, the presence and stage of disease, utilizing laboratory procedures, and performs autopsies to determine the nature and extent of disease, cause of death and effects of treatment.

10. Pediatrician: A physician who plans and carries out medical programs for children from birth through adolescence to aid in mental and physical growth and development.

11. Psychiatrist: A physician who studies, diagnoses and treats diseases and disorders of the mind.

12. Radiologist: A physician who diagnoses and treats diseases of the human body using X-rays and radioactive substances.

13. Surgeon: A physician who performs surgical treatment to correct deformities, repair injuries, prevent diseases and improve function in patients.

14. Urologist: A physician who diagnoses and treats diseases and disorders of the genito-urinary organs and tract.

Medications, care of. Some dentists keep medications in their offices. These should be kept out of the patient's sight and in a location where they cannot possibly be removed from the office by patients.

Memory aids

A hidden storage place should be maintained for narcotics, since physicans' and dentists' offices have been broken into by addicts or others seeking drugs.

Any staff member who shows an unusual interest in drugs of any kind should be brought to the attention of the physician. A variety of drugs may be abused, so a discrepancy in the supply of any drug whatsoever must be reported to the physician.

No assistant should ever take medication or remove it from his or her employer's office without the specific permission of the doctor.

Memory aids. A dental auxiliary or office manager with a good memory can be a tremendous asset to her employer. You can train yourself to have a better memory than you have now. Here are some suggestions:

1. Write down any items you must remember. By doing so you clear your mind of these things, thereby relieving you of the worry that you will forget them. Your mind is then free to concentrate on other things.

2. If a patient tells you personal details, such as names of his or her family, jot them down on his or her card. Then, when you see him or her again you can ask, "How are Bob and Betty?" because their names are there.

3. Make lists of the things you have to do (as suggested in the entry "Increasing Efficiency") again with the purpose of clearing your mind.

4. Concentrate on remembering patient's names:

   a. Look at, and think about the person. What color are his or her eyes? What color is his or her hair? How is it styled? How is the person dressed? Find something about that person that is memorable, and that you can link to his name.

   b. Say the name each time you speak to the person. Repetition helps one to remember.

5. If necessary, use a Polaroid photo attached to the patient's card to assist you in recalling who he or she is.

6. If you cannot photograph the patient, write a memo for yourself describing him or her. You may decide he looks like your Uncle George. Write that on the record in pencil.

7. Memory experts claim you can improve your memory by associating names with objects (e.g. for a person named Baker you would create a mental picture of Mr. Baker—obviously—baking a cake). When a name can be so linked, this process is easily used. However, with most names this is very difficult.

8. Look for other ways which help you to remember. By putting your mind to it, it has been proven that you can really improve in this important area. It can make a big difference in the attitude of the patients your doctor treats.

Merck Manual.   One of the best references, and one that you will probably find in your office, is called *"The Merck Manual."* It appeared first in 1899, and has increased in value year by year. It is not published each year, however. The publisher is **Merck, Shapp and Dohme Research Laboratories,** a division of Merck and Co., Inc., Rahway, NJ.

Actually its stated purpose is to provide useful information to practicing physicians; you, too, will find it extremely valuable.

The information provided in this book is current and accurate. There are 24 sections in the latest edition, the thirteenth, including a section on Dental & Oral Disorders.

Illnesses are covered in regard to etiology (cause), epidemiology (method of spreading of symptoms and signs), complications, diagnosis, prognosis, prophylaxis and treatment. While no personnel other than the doctor should ever treat a patient, the background information concerning illnesses can be helpful to the competent assistant. It can also assist the secretary in writing up reports and correspondence.

There are a variety of guides in the last chapter which also furnish information you may require, such as clinical and laboratory procedures.

Mercury, Monitoring to avoid overexposure.   Mercury is certainly one of your basic supplies. In its liquid form it is not hazardous, but when it vaporizes it becomes dangerous because it is quickly absorbed by the body, going into the bloodstream. If you are constantly exposed to it, the air you breathe should be carefully monitored, because the nervous system, the red corpuscles, the liver and the kidneys may be affected.

The **American Dental Associations Council on Dental Materials** recommends that periodic mercury-level determinations be done in each dental operatory. (**The Occupational Safety and OSHA Health Administration** has set a limit of 0.1 milligram per cu meter.)

Biotrol, Inc. 421 West 900 North Street, P.O. Box 556, Beneficial Industrial Park, North Salt Lake, UT 84054 (1-801-298-0880), has a mercury control system which includes information and a number of products which they have developed to control the mercury used, such as *Merclean Liquid Control*.

A monitoring system should certainly be used. A device may be worn or placed in the operatory as an area monitor. After a period of exposure it is returned to the company for analysis and a report is returned to you.

Metric system of weights and measures.

Weight:

1 milligram = 1,000 micrograms
1 gram = 1,000 milligrams
1 kilogram = 1,000 grams

Volume:

1 cubic centimeter = 1,000 cubic millimeters
1 liter = 1,000 cubic centimeters

Microfilming records. It is necessary to retain patient records for a variety of reasons:

1. In the event that the patient returns to the doctor he or she has a record of all treatment having been given.
2. In the event of litigation.
3. To fulfill regulations.

Because it is impossible to tell when records will be needed, most dentists keep them for periods over 10 years. One way in which this can be done without an inordinate waste of space is by microfilming those records which are considered inactive.

126

Microfilming is best done by a commercial organization which specializes in working on dental records. It would, of course, be necessary for your employer to make the decision of whether or not to adopt this system. However, it might be worthwhile for you to gather the information; this would include an approximation of the number of records in the inactive file, the space they take up, your present need of space and the cost of the procedure. The more information you can gather, the more informed will be your employer's decisions.

Music, background. Music in the background can serve a very important function. It can calm the nervous patient and make him or her less apprehensive. Music may be heard in the waiting room or throughout the office, in whatever rooms the doctor wishes it to be "piped." This can be done relatively easily with speakers placed in each room in which the music is desired.

The radio or tape recorder should be kept near the secretary's desk. If a system is being chosen, cassettes are probably superior to eight-tracks because the tapes last longer. A wide selection of both cassettes and eight-tracks are available from commercial record companies.

The secretary or assistant may be in charge of music. "Tunes" should come from an all-music radio station or from tapes. Records are too cumbersome and difficult to store for this purpose.

The type of music played depends on the doctor. It might reflect his or her musical preferences or those of the patients. If the choice is left up to the secretary, or possibly the assistant, then a "middle-of-the-road" type should be chosen. Disco and rock should both be avoided, unless the practice is devoted almost exclusively to young people. Show tunes and standards are considered to be good background music. Remember, though, not to play anything that may prove offensive.

Keep the volume down to the point where speech can be heard without the speaker having to shout above the music.

Music, individualized. Systems are now available that enable you to have music programs individualized to entertain your patients. In some respects these systems are similar to those offered on aircraft. The patient may select from one of several programs, and each patient may listen to his or her preferred program, through headphones. At each chair the patient has a small hand control and headset. The hand control enables the patient to choose the program and adjust the volume as well. The only item in each operatory is the headphone/hand control unit. One master control, which can be located anywhere in the office, controls up to 12 operatories. This master unit can also be shared by two or three separate offices. AM/FM programming can also be combined with the master unit to provide a fifth channel of programs to each operatory.

One company, **Novatone,** provides a music library of 24 hours of music and entertainment, and keeps your office constantly updated with a new four-hour program each month. For information contact **Audio Environments, NovaTone Division,** 900 East Pine Street, Seattle, WA 98122.

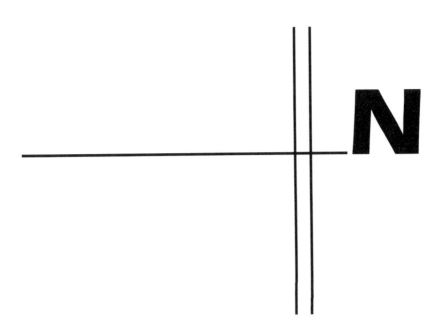

Narcotics. Prescribing, dispensing or administering drugs or narcotics is within the province of the practicing dentist and must be done according to federal and state regulations.

The Federal Food, Drug, and Cosmetic Act, passed originally in 1906, sought to control impure and adulterated food and drugs. Today, regulations deal also with "controlled substances" as a result of the passage of the Comprehensive Drug Abuse Prevention and Control Act. This act is concerned with the registration and control of the manufacture, distribution and dispensing of these controlled substances. Some of the more familiar of these are opiates such as heroin and morphine, amphetamines, and hallucinogens such as lysergic acid and products of the coca leaf. Many different drugs within each of those categories may be found in the doctor's supply closet (under lock and key, of course).

Laws and statutes vary from state to state. It is important for all personnel working in a dental office to be familiar with the regulations within their state. A dentist (or members of the staff) who fails to comply with the law may lose his or her license to practice dentistry. It is necessary to have a federal narcostics registry number from the Treasury Department, and possibly a state registry number as well, in order to prescribe controlled substances. It is entirely possible that your office may be visited by narcotics officers. Should this occur, be sure to ask for proper identification. (If you are still in doubt, telephone the office from which they claim to have been sent to be sure they are not impostors.) They are entitled to check the records kept by the doctor.

It is the job of the dental secretary or assistant to record on the patient's file any and all prescriptions given to that patient. Pharmacists are required to keep all of the prescriptions they fill and are accountable for their stocks of narcotics.

Prescription pads must be kept under lock and key and never within reach of patients in an office or examining room. If they are stolen, the theft should be reported to the police department. The use of a prescription by a person other than a physician or dentist is illegal. Even a professional, such as a psychologist, cannot prescribe drugs.

All drugs should be stored carefully and the place in which they are kept should be locked at all times. Even drug samples should be placed in a safe spot.

Certain drugs have a shelf life beyond which they should not be used. When this time has expired, the drugs should be destroyed so that no one can take them accidentally.

In dealing with narcotics, the integrity and honesty of the office personnel is critically important. If you notice that there are narcotics or prescription pads missing, you must inform your employer immediately. Reporting the loss is urgent because, as stated above, a physician may lose his or her license because of it. Everyone must be suspected if drugs or prescription pads are missing, and the guilty person must be found.

It is the doctor's decision as to where the narcotics are to be kept in his office. Once having established this, the doctor must depend on the staff for full and total cooperaton in this very important area.

National Children's Dental Health Month. Held annually, this event offers the opportunity to call attention to the need for dental care for all children. It offers an opportunity for your office to be of service to your community as well as excellent public relations.

Materials may be obtained by writing to the **Bureau of Health, Education and Audiovisual Services, American Dental Association,** 211 East Chicago Avenue, Suite 1648, Chicago, Illinois 60611. Usually these materials are very attractive as well as being extremely useful.

Your employer should be consulted in regard to whether he or she wishes to speak to youngsters. Generally, schools are happy to cooperate in dental health campaigns. You can assist by telephoning the schools and making arrangements.

An excellent practice builder, particularly for the newly established office, is the offer of dental examinations at no charge or at a reduced rate.

New home-care products.

Perio-aid. These are toothpick holders which enable the patient to remove plaque and massage the gingival areas. By holding toothpicks securely at the proper angle, *Perio-aid* allows the patient to effectively maintain difficult interproximal spaces, and helps the patient to reach normally inaccessible areas, such as the furcation area of the root.

Available from **Marquis Dental Manufacturing Company,** 15370 H Smith Road, Aurora, CO 80011.

Floss pik. This is a specially made device that resembles a cheese slicer because a small amount of floss is stretched between two sides of the holder. Using this pik the patient is able to clean and polish areas which are difficult to reach, and stimulate the gums as well.

Available from **Abba International Trade Company,** PO Box 110, Franklin, MI 48025.

Sonic scrub and Plak-Check. The *Sonic Scrub* is an ultrasonic denture cleaner, available to your patients. This device is easy to operate and affordable. Your denture wearers who are heavy smokers may be very happy to hear about this device, which has been shown to be very effective.

Plak-Check, a plaque detection system for home use is available. It consists of a yellow disclosing solution and a detection light. With this a patient is easily able to determine whether he or she is removing all the plaque which accumulates during the course of a day. The cost is very nominal, and for the patient who is very concerned about dental health, this is a valuable adjunct to home care.

Available from **Clairol,** PO Box 14207, Baltimore, MD 21268.

Denture bath. The L & R Denture Bath is a small inexpensive machine which is battery powered and very simple to use. It uses roto-sonic action, and is designed for everyday use. It's available at very reasonable prices from **L & R Manufacturing Company,** 577 Elm Street, Kearny, NJ 07032.

Floxite mirrors. These mirrors developed for home use have focused beams of light, so that the patient is able to see the area of his or her mouth which he or she is flossing. The mirror/light is useful for other purposes as well—such as putting on make-up, or examining one's eyes or ears.

Available from **Floxite Company, Inc.,** Niagara Falls, NY 14303.

New patients, obtaining.

New patient providers. This is a service that offers the name and addresses of selected people located in any area you select, printed on self-stick labels which can easily be applied to envelopes, practice newsletters, and informative brochures. You can easily send your message into the areas or communities where you would most like to expand your practice.

You may wish to reach any of the following: Families with children under 12, heads of households in the following age groups: 35 or younger, 36-45, 46-55, 56-64, all ages, 64 and younger, 65 and older. You may also wish to reach people who have recently moved into your area.

For information contact **New Patient Providers,** 4849 Golf Road, Suite 400, Skokie, IL. 60077.

You may set up a standing order to receive names on a monthly basis.

Market area analysis. A report taken from the U.S. Census is available which gives you population by ethnic group and age, household data, marital and family data, education and occupation, mobility data and key 1983 estimates.

In an urban practice, a radius analysis of a one, two or three mile area is standard. In a rural or suburban practice, a zip code analysis is recommended.

A plan to assist you in using the data is also included.

This service is available from **Judy Turks & Associates, Inc.,** 23151 Plaza Pointe Drive, Suite 120, Laguna Hills, CA 92653.

Also available from this group is a catalog showing sophisticated dental practice ads, called "Ad Helper for Dentists." Over 50 ads are included. The ads are priced at a fraction of what it would cost if you hired an advertising agency to custom design them. With any ad, purchase information on how to run your advertisign campaign is included.

Practice Resource Institute. This division of **Semantodontics, Inc.** (3714 East Indian School Road, Phoenix, AZ 85018) works on the premise "20 percent of dentists are getting 80 percent of the new patients." It assists the dental staff in developing referral sources, by teaching them the specific techniques necessary to stimulate practice growth. Seminars are offered on such topics as living with stress successfully, teamwork, and staff effectiveness; they include *Beyond the Basics* and *Super Duper Auxiliary Seminars* which are conducted year-round throughout the country, biannually in Maui, Hawaii, and Seminars-at-Sea in the Caribbean and Mediterranean.

A monthly newsletter (*Practice Smart*) introduces new concepts and products. All areas of **Semantodontics** stress the people-to-people approach in dentistry.

New patient's records: the personal history. Certain information is needed regarding every patient. This information may be obtained orally if you have a private area available. Do not, however, ask questions where you may be overheard. Patients are embarrassed if their private affairs are discussed where they are no longer confidential.

It will save you time if a duplicated sheet is prepared which you can hand to the patient for him or her to fill out, and this procedure also insures privacy.

New products

The information to be included is as follows:

Name: Last   First   Middle

Address:

Telephone number at home:

Name of spouse:

If not married, check:

        single ___   widowed ___   divorced ___

Occupation:

Place of employment:

Insurance company:

Place this sheet on the doctor's desk before he or she sees the patient.

The medical record: This portion of the patient's record may be taken by the hygienist, the office manager, the assistant or by the doctor. This is entirely a matter of preference, and is entirely at the discretion of the dentist. See *Medical History*.

New products to call to the attention of your doctor.

Models—TMJ Internal Derangement Model. This model enables the doctor to show the patient the exact nature of the joint problem, and the basis for his or her treatment of it. The model even "clicks" when the jaws are open. Many conditions can be shown by using it.

Models such as manikins, flossing/brushing models, large toothbrushes, and rubber dentoform models (from which demonstration models may be made from stone or plaster) are also available from **Columbia Dentoform Corp.,** 49 East 21st Street, New York NY 10010.

Emergency Insurance Drug Kit. This kit contains a variety of drugs, plus the symptoms for which they should be given.

The kit is color coded so that it is easy to see all of this at a glance. For example, Vasopressors are indicated to give for a rapid fall in blood pressure, anti-allergic drugs to combat undue reactions to medication or to combat severe asthmatic attack, stimulants to combat respiratory depression.

Available from **Healthfirst Corporation,** Box 279, Edwards, WA 98020.

There is an optional automatic-refill program which assures the freshness and effectiveness of the drugs in the kit. Since this program is automatic, drugs are sent to you when necessary, and you need not keep track of this.

Blood pressure and pulse rate computers. The computer-controlled performance of *Medipulse* equipment represents the new technology available for the taking of blood pressure and pulse rate. Both of these are taken in a little more than one-half minute.

Medipulse 313 gives a printout, showing date, time, systolic pressure, diastolic pressure and pulse rate. The instrument may be battery or AC operated. It has automatic inflation and deflation.

Other models are available as well, with different capabilities, such as manual inflation, and automatic deflation. For information write to **Somatronix Research Corporation,** PO Box 919, 240 Main Street, Bristol, CT 06010.

Tray setups. Are tray setups used in your office? A variety of stainless steel or plastic trays, with spaces for instruments and burs, plus color-coding tapes as well as racks and cabinets are available. From **Dencraft,** PO Box 47, Moorestown, NJ 08057.

Bib Bin. An acrylic countertop towel dispenser, "Bib Bin," which holds approximately 75 towels, is an attractive way to have them at your disposal. Available from **Interstate Drug Exchange, Inc.**, Engineers Hill, Plainview, NJ 11803.

Anti-static spray. **Evans** *Anti-static spray* is a product which prevents the build-up of static electricity. It's clean and will not stain, so it may be used on all surfaces, including clothing, where static electricity builds up.

Available from **Evans Specialty Company, Inc.**, 14 East 15th Street, POB 24189, Richmond, VA 23224.

Evans also can supply you with a "Statkleer Computer Cloth" for cleaning the CRT screen of your computer, thereby eliminating static video interference.

Automatic processing for intraoral x-ray film. The *Philips 410* is the equipment which does just this. Since the process is automatic, dry-to-dry x-rays are availabe in six and one half minutes, whereas wet readings require only three minutes. Furthermore, no special plumbing installation is necessary, and the processor takes up less than two feet of space, is one foot wide and less than one foot high.

Available from **Philips Medical Systems,** 102 Commerce Road, Stamford, CT 06902.

Cutting costs of forms. *Make Your Own forms Using Your Office Copier* contains 78 ready-to-use masters of forms used every day. Available from **Caddylak Systems,** 201 Montrose Road, Westbury, NY 11590.

Dental Insurance Directory. This publicaton, available for your geographic area, contains specific information for each company, such as the annual maximums, annual deductibles, fee schedules, eligibility requirements and the fiscal year of the plan. The company the patient works for is listed and the company that insures them. You're shown to whom and where to send the form, as well as the date of eligibility, the starting date of the fiscal year and family eligibility. You can tell a patient exactly what his or her insurance covers, and immediately establish a payment schedule for the "out-of-pocket" portion of the fee. The material is updated on a yearly basis to insure accuracy.

Directories are available from **Dental Insurance Services, Inc.**, PO Box 485, Belmont, MA 02178.

Newspaper column. One excellent way for your office to be advertised is through columns that your office supplies, and that are printed in your local newspaper. Of course there is a cost for the space, but the rewards can be far in excess of that cost. The column, which should appear weekly for maximum effect, should contain information of value to the patient, and be written on a ninth-grade reading level, so that the majority of potential patients reading it are able to understand it. (If your target population is of less education, then it is important to keep the material within their framework of understanding.)

Columns, of course, must be carefully written. This may be done by your employer, if he or she has the time and inclination to do so. If not, and if there is a capable member of the staff who can do this, then that person can handle the chore.

The question-and-answer type of column is good for many reasons, among them the fact that it is easily read, and research has shown that more people are inclined to read that format than they are to read straight narrative writing.

The column may contain "chatty" information about patients, about the staff and the neighborhood, if desired, or it may be strictly informational or a combination of the two.

It is possible to purchase material of the informative nature already produced, "ghost written" so to speak.

One source of the commercial columns available is **Dental Dialogue, Inc.**, 309 West 7th Avenue, Columbus, OH 43201. Written by Dr. Herb Urell and Linda Urell, it consists of questions (and answers); some of the typical questions are "Is it true that the fluoride in toothpaste can be lost when it gets too old?" or "I am told that if you can avoid it, you should never lose any tooth in your mouth. Why?"

Many dentists are already using this type of publicity, which is educational and highly professional.

Nitrous oxide, Monitoring to avoid overexposure.   If nitrous oxide is used in your office, it is possible you are being overexposed to it. There is the possibility that even very small (trace) amounts may cause a danger to the health of the entire staff.

Such conditions as hepatic disease, renal disease and disorders of the central nervous system may result. If a female member of the dental staff is overexposed, it may result in spontaneous abortion or congenital abnormalities in children. This fact was brought out in a study by Cohen, Brown, Wu, et al, written up in the *Journal of the ADA,* July 1980 issue.

There is a monitor now available which enables you to check the N_2O concentration in your dental office. It is used once every three months, and the method for its use is extremely simple. The monitor is can shaped; the can is opened in the area to be monitored and after a short exposure period it is resealed and returned. An analysis is done and sent back to you. Clip badges may be used instead of the aforementioned monitor.

For further information contact **Siemens Gammasonics, Health Physics Services,** 2000 Nuclear Drive, Des Plaines, II, 60018.

Non-English–speaking patients. It is crucial that the doctor be able to understand patients when they describe their symptoms. You are in a position to be of assistance in this regard.

If, upon interviewing a new patient, you discover a problem in communication, request the patient to bring in someone who is able to act as an interpreter. If there is some urgency, this person may translate for the patient on the telephone. However, the doctor should be able to fully understand exactly what the patient is trying to get across.

If you are working in an area where a language other than English predominates, it is worthwhile for you to learn enough of that language to be able to communicate with patients. It appears the United States is becoming bilingual, with Spanish as a second language, and if your office is in an area where knowledge of that language is necessary, learn what you need to know. This would include numbers, parts of the body and simple courtesies. People react very positively when a staff member uses their language, even for something as simple as "How are you?"

Non-English–speaking patients are often frightened by the language barrier they experience. Reassuring them should be part—an important part—of your work, and if you are able to do so in their language, it is particularly effective.

Keep a phrase book handy if you find you run into language problems frequently. It can take some of the mystery out of the situation.

Be aware, too, that persons speaking only a little English often make errors, so, again, it is advisable to be very cautious. Where the problem is a serious one, great care should be taken.

Nonverbal communication. Everyone of us communicates without saying a word, and this nonverbal communication may make a big difference with your patients.

What are the best ways to communicate nonverbally? Probably the key word is *Smile.* A welcoming smile says more than many words, if the words are spoken hurriedly or offhandedly. The expression on your face can make a patient feel good about coming to the office, or it can do just the opposite. Remember that many patients are afraid when they walk into the office, and need that extra support which you can offer. Begin by smiling.

Next, if possible, take the patient's hand or touch his or her arm to further show warmth and support.

Do not give the patient the idea that you are so busy you have no time for him or her. This can have a disastrous effect, again because people are very vulnerable when coming for dental work.

When you have financial matters to discuss, or anything else of a confidential nature, make sure that those words are spoken quietly and in a soft voice. Imagine how you would feel if you said, in a loud tone, "Your bill is four hundred dollars." Even though you may not be accusing the patient of not wanting to pay, he or she may get that idea.

When you are assisting at the chair, many patients are comforted if you take their hands and hold them. Also, while the doctor is working on the patient, if you frown or look serious, it is easy for the patient to think something has gone wrong, and become worried needlessly. Frequent eye contact is good because it, too, is reassurance, as is, of course, the smile.

As you do any work involving the patient or instruments used to treat him or her, do it with care and precision, so that the person sitting in that chair feels you know what you are doing, and since you are taking good care of these inanimate objects, you will take good care of him or her too.

Several other factors are nonverbal communicators. For example, if your uniform is not spotless and pressed, you present a messy image, which is to be avoided. The same is true of

Nosebleed

any type of odor. If you have a problem with bad breath or body odor, it is very important that you take steps to avoid these. You are in very close contact with people, and you have to be doubly careful to present the image you wish to present, and not a negative one which says, in effect, "I really don't care about the way I present myself."

Nosebleed. There are many causes of nosebleeds. Numerous small blood vessels supply the nasal tissues. These have thin walls that are easily broken, causing nosebleeds, when they are damaged by blows to the nose. High blood pressure may cause these small vessels to break or they may be broken from irritation.

To stop a nosebleed, with the doctor's approval, use the following procedures:

1. The patient must be able to breath through his or her mouth. To make this easier, the patient should be seated, with the head bent slightly forward.
2. Have the patient hold his or her nose pinched closed for 15 minutes.
3. Then, release slowly so that if a clot has formed it will not be disturbed. The patient should be warned not to blow the nose because this may disturb the clot that has been formed.
4. If bleeding has not stopped, place a cold cloth or ice on the nose and face. This may stop the bleeding by constricting the blood vessels.

The doctor should be notified whether or not bleeding persists.

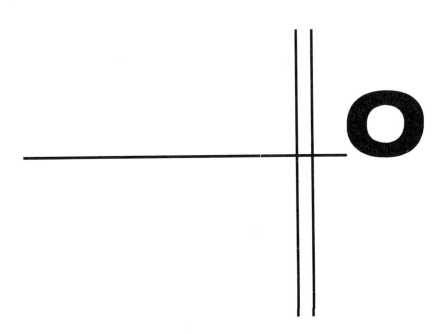

Observing patient behavior. This is one more way in which you, as a dental auxiliary or office manager, can be of help to your employer.

In every office there are patients who need reassurance because of their nervousness. They may not "open up" to the doctor as they do to a staff member. If the information they offer you is pertinent, it should be referred to the doctor. Otherwise, if the patient has been calmed down sufficiently this should not be necessary.

Patients often need reassurance and support. Many may fear anesthesia more than the actual dental work. If you observe a patient who appears worried, try to learn exactly what it is he or she is afraid of. For some it is being allergic to drugs, or reacting negatively to being anesthetized. For others it is that they will talk too freely under anesthetic. Reassure them, in all cases. For example, tell them they are watched carefully for signs of allergy or negative reactions.

Odors. One of the most distinctive odors in the world is that of oil of cloves (eugenol) which is always associated with dental offices. By eliminating it, you can also get rid of the negative feelings engendered in many patients—patients who are already feeling anxious about visiting the dentist.

Commercial deodorizers, some using only one small drop, can remove much of that characteristic smell.

As a dental assistant, who comes into close contact with people, you may want to use a light perfume or cologne. That may possibly help to distract a nervous patient, and will make your own personal environment more pleasant. Avoid anything heavy or overly sweet, because such scents would negate what you are trying to do.

Office mailboxes. In order to get messages to staff members quickly and without disturbing routines, a system of "mailboxes" may be set up. In this case the mailbox may be any receptable which belongs to an individual, and where mail or messages may be placed. This is a definite help to the receptionist, who, having placed a message in the box is no longer responsible for it. The responsibility for checking it falls to the staff member herself.

However, the doctor's personal mail and messages should be placed on his or her desk. This rule applies to all of the doctors in the practice (if this is a multiple practice).

This system is used in many schools, in order to expedite the distribution of mail to the staff members.

Should there be emergency messages, these should, of course, be called to the attention of the person involved. The person taking the calls should not consider all calls from the children of staff members as emergencies—unless they legitimately are.

Office maintenance. The dental auxiliaries are responsible for the maintenance of the office. Since a dental office must be as "spic and span" as is humanly possible, this is an important part of their responsibilities. They should supervise the work of a cleaning service, or private person, who is engaged to do the heavy cleaning once a week. This would include the following:

Washing and polishing vinyl floors

Vacuuming rugs

Cleaning windows

Dusting and polishing furniture and woodwork

Polishing all metal surfaces

Cleaning venetian blinds

On a daily basis, the following must be attended: (A part-time employee may take over these functions.)

Dusting all furniture

Dust mopping all floors except those that are carpeted

Wiping examination tables and cabinets

Arranging the contents of cabinet drawers, and noting when supplies must be ordered

Emptying waste baskets

Arranging magazines

Adjusting shades

Watering plants

Once every three months, there are other maintenance procedures which should be followed:

Polishing all white cabinets, examination tables, etc. using special polishes to keep them white

Removing the content of all shelves, and polishing the interiors of cabinets

Removing glass covers on desks and tables, and polishing both sides

Wiping plastic furniture

Washing Venetian blinds

Vacuuming drapes

Checking magazines, and discarding old issues

Washing the insides of waste baskets

Office manager's manual of procedures. The following are the basic tasks usually performed by the office manager:

1. Morning routines associated with opening the office
2. Greeting and speaking with patients
3. Scheduling patients
4. Preparing the Day Sheet
5. Billing and collection
6. Paying bills
7. Filing

8. Supervising the housekeeping care of the office
9. Filling out insurance forms
10. Keeping records of all financial transactions
11. Handling correspondence
12. Advertising for and screening job applicants
13. Evening routines associated with closing the office
14. Responsibilities relevant to the doctor's personal or business affairs

Office manager—signed letters. There is some mail which can go out over your signature, thereby saving the doctor's time.

Several titles are possible. Ask your doctor how he wishes the outgoing mail be signed. The following are possibilities:

May June, Office Manager

May June, Business Manager

Since all outgoing mail is written on the doctor's letterhead, either of these signatures is appropriate. "May June," however, with no further explanation, would be very bad policy.

Office newsletter. The newsletter is a device that fosters communication between the dental office and patients. It may be sent out whenever the doctor desires to do so, or at specific times during the year.

Usually newsletters are printed on $8\frac{1}{2} \times 11''$ paper, folded in three parts to form a small brochure. They may contain any article the doctor feels will be of benefit to his or her patients, as well as a personal message to them.

This is a good method of bringing important information to patients, such as word of new techniques and new medication; it also serves to convey personal information, and news of the office and its hours and routines. You can obtain material by reading and summarizing articles in dental journals and health publications, or the doctor may prefer to write his own material. Commercial newsletters are another possibility.

Opening the office in the morning. The office manager or the dental assistant should arrive at least fifteen minutes to one-half hour before any patient is scheduled.

You should determine the amount of time you generally need, and allow for that. If you can get everything necessary for the preparation of the day accomplished beforehand, the entire day will go smoothly. Much of this can be done at the end of the day before.

The tasks that must be done before seeing patients include:

1. Setting up the waiting room. This includes dusting the tops of tables, straightening up the magazines, and emptying and washing the ash trays.
2. Telephoning the answering service to get any messages which were left, and making any necessary telephone calls resulting from these messages.
3. Preparing the day sheet (see entry) for each consultation and examining room.
4. Selecting the patient records and putting them in place on the doctor's desk.
5. Checking for the mail—if delivery is early in your community.

By the time the first patient arrives, you should be settled down and ready to greet them.

Oral hygiene instruction. If your employer does not use a dental hygienist, it may become part of your duties to provide oral hygiene instruction, a valuable service, to the patient. If so, you must be ready to field questions and explain the techniques in a readily understandable manner, and actively encourage and aid the patient.

This is part of the preventative aspect of modern dental practice, one that is geared to intercept dental disease before it takes place. Remember that teaching adequate dental hygiene involves the formation of positive daily habits and may be extremely difficult to achieve.

The brushing technique your doctor endorses may vary. Whether it involves horizontal or vertical strokes of the brush is

145

secondary in importance to how effectively the teeth are cleaned. Any method that works and is easy for the patient will do. What the dental assistant must stress is brushing the area at the gumline where the tissue is not attached to the tooth. The bristles of the toothbrush must be directed at a 45° angle to this area. A study model with this critical area outlined in colored ink can be very helpful. An oversized toothbrush and dental model is helpful in this regard as well.

Flossing instructions should be done in front of a mirror. You may choose to have the patient watch you floss their teeth, initially. Disclosing solution, which stains plaque and debris, is a valuable adjunctive aid that enables the patient to see areas needing attention. Floss should be wound around the fingers until only an inch and a half is available to be placed between the teeth. The patient should be alerted to the hazards of snapping the floss into the gum too forcefully. Once threaded through the contact, it should be wrapped around the tooth and by use of a shoe shining-type motion, brought back through the contact. As the floss is saturated, it may be unwound and a fresh area used. Every contact area has two surfaces to be cleaned except the distal of the third molar. Flossing should be done at home in front of a mirror, and it is helpful to have the patient divide the teeth into four quadrants.

Special devices are commercially available to floss under bridgework or in the exposed furcation of molars.

If you indeed find yourself performing this service for your patients, remember that the teaching of these skills is as valuable a service to the patient as those provided by anyone in the office, including the dentist.

OSHA (Occupational Safety and Health Act). The law often referred to as OSHA protects employees in all businesses including dental offices. An employer must provide a work place free from hazards.

Under the jurisdiction of the **United States Department of Labor,** OSHA establishes standards to protect workers on the job. Since each state has its own safety laws, it is necessary for you to contact the state office for information if you feel you have a problem. It is not necessary for one's health or safety to be jeopardized because of any situation "on the job."

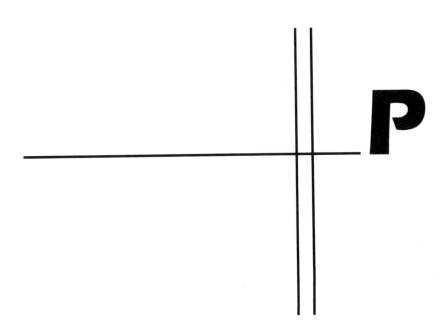

Part-time help. There are times in the year when assistance is needed—and for which part-time help is ideally suited.

"Part-timers" should be hired for no more than 19 hours per week. In this way the office payroll is kept down because they do not receive the same fringe benefits as full-time help.

Part-timers are valuable because they can do seasonal work, such as the addressing and sending out of Christmas cards. They can do clean-up work and be trained to substitute for other staff members when the latter are absent.

In hiring part-timers, it is advisable to have the office manager do the interviewing and subsequently help with the training. Part-timers should be made to feel welcome, and should be told, specifically, what work they will be doing. In that way disappointments and false expectations may be avoided, and the time spent in training will not be wasted.

A well-trained part-timer who is available to come in when other staff members are absent can be a great asset to the smooth operation of a busy office. If she is trained in all areas she can step in wherever and whenever she is needed.

Patient education. You may often be asked to explain work your dentist is planning to do, or has already done. Charts are

Patient's financial record keeping

available that enable you to do so—providing, of course, your employer agrees that you may do so.

One chart, for example, shows a sectioned primary lower molar, with other illustrations of primary and permanent teeth, and also shows proper tooth-brushing and flossing techniques.

Models are also available from **Anatomical Chart Company,** 7124 Clark Street, Chicago, IL 60626.

Patient's financial record keeping. The patient's financial files may be kept in a variety of ways:

1. Index Cards—A 5 × 7″ index card file may be set up, and arranged alphabetically.

2. Large folders—A larger form may be used which can be kept in a looseleaf binder, or in a filing cabinet. Commercial forms are available for this purpose.

3. The information which is necessary includes the following (on top of card):

Patient's name, last name first:

Address:

Telephone number:

Person to be billed:

(Type each column 1″)

Date	Nature of Visit	Charge	Form Submitted (Date)	Paid	Nature of Payment	Balance	Date Payment in Full

By using this format, it is easy to tell if a patient's account has been paid in full, or if there is money outstanding. All payments received should be posted the same day so that patients' accounts are up to date.

It is also simple to see how much money is outstanding at any time. In the column indicating nature of payment, the words, "Cash," "Check," "Insurance," etc. should be indicated.

In the column "Form Submitted," the date should be indicated. Often patients request this information; when placed on this record it is readily available.

Patient records, requested from another dentist. In order to obtain records or X-rays for a patient of yours from another doctor, a simple request such as the following, should be made:

Dear Dr. X:

Miss Mary Ann Smith of 1010 Battery Avenue, San Diego, California has requested treatment in our office.

We would appreciate it if you would send a copy of her records to us as soon as possile. If necessary, her X-rays may be substituted.

Sincerely yours,

_____

Where there may be a name change, it is wise to use full names. If Mary Ann Smith were to have become Mrs. it would be wise to use her married name, as well. (e.g. Mary Ann Smith (Mrs. John Stuart Smith) for proper identification.)

Patient records, to be sent to another doctor. In order to make this transfer, the patient must write a letter or note to your employer, requesting the transfer be made. Explain that this is office procedure, and that you will be pleased to comply with the request when it is made in this way.

A sample letter might be as follows:

Dear Dr. Smith:

Please transfer my records (or X-rays) to Dr. Joseph Jones, 1502 Haven Street, Chicago, Illinois, 60601. Since I have moved to that city, the transfer is necessary.

Thank you for your cooperation.

Sincerely,

Patient's signature

Paying bills

As soon as this notice is received, a copy of your records should be sent to Dr. Jones.

Always send records by Certified Mail, with a signed, returned receipt requested.

Paying bills.   All bills should be verified. Never pay a bill unless you are sure it is valid. This applies when the bill is for merchandise of any kind or for services.

Pay all bills by check (unless you are instructed to do otherwise by your employer) from the Business Account.

Checks should be recorded in the checkbook and in your Expenditures Book.

Determine, with your employer, the time when bills are to be paid. This may be as soon as they come in, at the first of the month, at the fifteenth of the month or the last week of the month.

If you are in charge of paying the doctor's personal bills, make sure the checks are written on the doctor's Personal Account.

Enclose all bills with the invoice which accompanied them. Save a portion of the bill showing the service or goods which were received for it.

It is entirely possible for duplicate bills to be sent to you; therefore, before paying any bills, check your Expenditures Book to be sure it has not been paid before.

Payment of fees.   Some dentists choose to discuss fees with patients, while others prefer to leave this discussion to the office manager. Another method is to bill the patient after each visit. Bills may also be presented as the patient leaves the office. When this is done it should be routine for the office manager to say, "The fee for your visit today was X dollars, Mrs. Smith. Would you like to pay it now to save you the bother of sending a check?"

If the latter procedure is followed, there must be some means of communication between you and the doctor. He or she may write the amount of the fee right on the patient's card which you can pick up at the end of the visit. Another method is to use a short form listing the date, the patient's name, the procedure done and the charge. The doctor may give this to the patient with instructions to hand it to you, or may place it on the desk from which you pick it up.

Behave in such a manner that the patient realizes he or she is expected to make a payment either at the conclusion of the appointment or soon thereafter.

Payroll deductions. Payroll deductions can include a number of things, but there are two deductions which are required by law.

One is the Federal Insurance Contributions Act (FICA), which established Social Security and the graduated deductions taken from every employee's pay. This amount paid by the employee must be matched by the employer when the funds are deposited to the federal government.

The second deduction is Federal Withholding Tax (FWT), the federal income tax deduction, which is also a graduated tax set by Congress. Other possible deductions taken from employees' salaries may include state and local taxes, health and accident insurance, pension funds, union dues, loans, charitable contributions and a plan to purchase U.S. Savings Bonds.

Periodicals and newsletters. These should be placed on the doctor's desk, underneath all other correspondence. After reviewing them, he or she may place them in the file box, or discard them. Have a large wastepaper basket easily available for this purpose.

Personal appearance. The personal appearance of the dental office staff and the appearance of the office convey an impression that remains with the patient long after he or she has left the office. It goes without saying that everything must be spotlessly clean. A musty, dusty appearance is very bad for the image the doctor is trying to create.

In regard to your appearance, whether or not you will wear a uniform will depend entirely on the doctor for whom you work. He or she may decide that the hygienist and the assistant should wear one, but the office manager need not. Or, the entire staff may be in uniform.

Secondly, your doctor may decide the uniforms should be a color other than white.

Personalizing the office

Uniforms must be spotless, and also wrinklefree. Simple jewelry may be worn, but not ornate pieces, or long, dangling earrings.

Your shoes, if you are wearing a white uniform, should be white as well. However, they should be shoes, and not sandals, or play shoes of any kind. Very high heels are out of place, as well. Your shoes should be comfortable, and enable you to do all the walking you must do without annoyance.

No person working in a dental office should be so made up that she looks as if she should be on the stage. Appropriate daytime makeup is acceptable. Your hair should not be "fly-away" or messy. It should be tied back, if it is very long, so that the overall impression is of neatness.

Excessively long fingernails are also out of place in a dental office. Your hands should look cared for, and the nails, if polished, should not appear chipped. If you must wash your hands several times a day, it is advisable to have a bottle of hand lotion, or a hand cream available, and use it several times a day to avoid chapping and cracking. **Neutrogenia Norwegian Formula Hand Cream** is excellent for this purpose.

Personalizing the office. All patients want to be treated as individuals. It is important to call patients by name, once they have given you that information. If the name is difficult to pronounce, write it phonetically next to the correct spelling.

Every staff member should listen carefully to what patients tell them. Jot down personal information such as the person's occupation, the names of his or her children and his or her hobbies or interests. You will then be able to refer to this when you see the patient again.

When a patient wishes to talk, it is important that he or she be listened to. However, in a busy office one cannot spend too much time on this without falling behind. You can say, with a smile, "I've enjoyed speaking with you. Please excuse me. There's some work inside I must attend to now." Another way of handling this situation is to have another staff member call you away from the patient. As you leave you would, of course, apologize.

When you ask a patient to fill out a form, explain it carefully first. This will save you time as well as personalize the task.

Never lie to a patient. If necessary, of course you will be sympathetic, but do not say anything that will make the patient lose confidence in you.

The "Golden Rule" is the best piece of advice in the world in regard to personalizing your office; "Do unto others as you would have them do unto you."

Petty cash. This is cash kept on hand for daily use. An amount is decided upon by the doctor (usually approximately $25 to $50) and from this fund expenses of a minor nature are paid. The office manager is in charge of this money. Expenditures of this nature might include medications purchased from a local shop (rather than in bulk from the usual supplier), postage, electric bulbs and delivery charges. The cash transactions should be entered in an envelope in a place where it is accessible, such as a desk drawer or filing cabinet.

For each expenditure a voucher should be placed in the envelope immediately, so that none of the money is lost. It is certainly possible to use this fund and neglect to put in the voucher. If so, valuable time is spent trying to "find" the money.

On the voucher the amount spend should be written, plus the date, the purchase for which the money was used, and the signature of the person who spent the money. There are simple forms available for this purpose, or you can construct your own.

When the doctor takes money from petty cash, request he or she sign a slip, just as other personnel do.

Once a month, the fund should be replenished.

It is not a good policy for anyone to borrow from the petty cash fund. The temptation to do so is there, but should be avoided.

If you find there is a need to replenish the petty cash fund more than once a month, suggest to your employer that a larger amount be placed in the fund, so that his or her valuable time is not wasted on this.

Photocopying. The photocopier has become an essential tool of every efficient office. It can be used for a variety of tasks, including billing. This may be done by photocopying the patient's record, and mailing the copy which shows all charges and payments, as well as the balance due.

Duplicates of all correspondence which goes out of the office should be kept on file. If, after you have prepared a letter for the doctor's signature, he or she adds a comment, that should be kept on file. You may find it a money-saver to use carbon copies for ordinary mail, but whenever additions are made, photocopies should be made for the file.

Occasionally articles appear in newspapers that your doctor may wish to photocopy for certain patients.

If your doctor has a poor memory, and you give him or her memos, it is wise to keep a copy of these, as well, so that you may resubmit them immediately before they have to be acted upon.

When dealing with insurance forms, you will learn which companies consistently "lose" claim forms. If you then photocopy their forms before submitting them, you can save time later on when duplicates are requested.

When patients request their records be sent to another doctor or anywhere else, it is worthwhile to photocopy them before mailing them out since there is always the possibility of their getting lost in the mail.

Photography.   The dental assistant can be of great help to her employer if he or she requires photographs be taken, and the assistant can serve as photographer.

The best camera for this purpose is a single lens reflex, 35 mm. Some of the preferred manufactures are **Minolta, Nikon** or **Canon**.

Special lenses are required. A 90 mm. macro-lens enables the photographer to take excellent close-up photographs. (This is termed "one to one." "One to two" pictures are half life-size. This continues up to "one to ten," wherein the photograph is one tenth of life-size.)

There are two types of lights:

> *Ring light*—which consists of a ring around the lens, and is good for intraoral photography. It is useful for photographing small instruments at close range.

Point light—this is similar to a single beam—like a flashlight. It is useful for photographing full-face, for example.

The most appropriate film for use with these lights is *Ektachrome 64* . The lights can be varied; this is explained on the light source. They use regular 110 current, rather than batteries.

The slides which are taken may be used for lectures or patient education. Prints may be made from them easily.

If the doctor needs only full-face photography, the *Polaroid* cameras are excellent, and very simple to use.

To use any of this equipment effectively, the assistant must be trained. However, after learning the skill, the technique is not difficult.

Having "before and after" photographs of the quality of your employer's work, especially in these times of emphasis on "esthetic" dentistry, can be a huge practice builder. You should have any patient whom you want to use for this purpose sign a release to this effect, before taking or displaying their pictures. This can easily be done in a very flattering manner.

Plants. The presence of well-kept, living, green plants in the waiting room is a healthy sign. Patients react well to this type of stimulus.

Choose plants such as Swedish Ivy, which grows well and can easily be used as a source for more plants, simply by cutting off pieces and rooting them in water. Philodenrum, Pothos, English Ivy and Spider Plants also grow well with a minimum of care.

Spraying the plants with water daily keeps them looking fresh.

A flowering plant can add color to an otherwise drab office. Mums, for instance, last quite a few weeks and are bright and cheerful.

About once a month use a plant fertilizer to restore the mineral content of the soil.

You will find the plants will be "conversation pieces," and will more than justify their expense and care by the effect they have on the office.

Postage meter

If your office is in need of brightening, fresh-cut flowers can add color and attractiveness to it. They are, however, considerably more expensive than plants.

One staff member should be given the responsibility of caring for all of the plants in the office.

Postage meter. Available for every office, regardless of size, the postage meter eliminates the need for licking stamps. It also keeps foolproof records of postage expenses. The U.S. Postal Service licenses the meter. The machine itself may be purchased or rented. To buy postage, however, it must be taken to the post office, where it is set. The postage is paid for in advance.

The letters to be mailed are passed through the meter, and the postage is stamped directly on them.

Pouring models. An impression may be poured in plaster, or more commonly, in dental stone.

Dental stone is usually stored in a metal bin in the office laboratory, and mixed in a rubber bowl. A quantity of water is poured into the bowl, and stone is sifted into it until the water is saturated. It is then mixed with a spatula, and more stone is added and spatulated until a consistency similar to sour cream is reached. At this point either the rubber bowl should be vibrated on a special vibrator designed for this purpose, or the impression itself should be placed on the vibrator as stone is poured into the impression. If the latter technique is used, never place the impression itself, but only the tray handle, on the vibrator. Pour small quantities of stone into the impression from the back of the tray, filling the tooth spaces completely before adding stone to the soft tissue spaces. As stone flows into the impression, you will notice air bubbles rising on the surface of the stone. Keep vibrating or tapping the tray handle until all bubbles are gone. After the entire surface of the impression is covered with stone, make a patty of the remaining mixture, fit it over the impression, allow it to set for a few minutes, and trim the stone to the borders of the tray with a plaster knife.

A wet towel or newspaper should be placed in the tongue space of lower impressions before pouring to leave space between the base and the impression.

When completely set, the models may be trimmed and neatened on a lathe. Never invert a poured model until it is completely set.

Practice building. In building a practice it is important to know that "the office is a lengthened shadow of the doctor," and that it is his or her attitude and leadership which makes the difference. With strong, positive feelings and goals for growth, successful practice building can be achieved. The work of the dental auxiliaries is extremely important in accomplishing this. All of the suggestions made here are worthy of your consideration.

The care and nurture of patients is basic.

1. Every patient wishes to feel important, and every person working in the dental office must keep this in mind. How can we do this? First, the patient should be greeted with smiles and cheerful words by the entire staff. Nothing is worse than a gloomy dental office.

2. The secretary should keep note of the patient's personal life—job, family, and interests. Jot these down on his or her card—so that the doctor and assistant can say, "How's Jackie doing in college?" or "How's your golf game doing?" Questions like there are very impressive and delight patients.

3. Touch patients. Dental assistants should be trained to put a hand on the patient's arm, and to be warm and reassuring. This is especially necessary when a patient is in the dental chair—and is frightened. If the assistant holds a patient's hand and is reassuring, the patient remembers this. Another thing the assistant can do when a patient is frightened is to make a special effort to take his or her mind off the work at hand by engaging the patient in conversation which is meaningful. Chatting about the weather won't do it, but taking note of the patient's personal affairs and speaking about them will.

4. After every major dental appointment, a phone call by the office manager to the patient can do much to make the patient feel very important. (If scheduling permits, this type of call may also be made by the dental assistant.) The time invested is relatively short, but the effect on the patient is well worth the effort. Just a pleasant, albeit simple, "This is Mary Jones, of Dr. Smith's office. How are you feeling today?" will impress even the most cynical person.

Practice building

Get patients to refer.   One of the best sources of patients is through referrals. Any member of the dental office staff, but usually the office manager, should say the following: "Many patients ask us if we are accepting new patients. We want you to know that we certainly are—and we thank you for your referrals."

Once a patient refers someone, it is absolutely essential that that patient be acknowledged, and thanked. This is the responsibility of the office manager. A card, flowers, a small gift—any of these are appropriate. Do note the importance of this step. Satisfied patients can be walking advertisements for your office.

Pedodontics—how to build a young practice.   If you are anxious to build up your dental practice, treating children may be one way to do so. There are certain techniques that will help in this regard.

1. Explanations to the child by either the office manager or the dental assistant are important. Explain to the child exactly what dental work is going to be done. Assure children that it will not hurt, if indeed it will not. (Never say it won't if the treatment might be painful.)

2. Present the child with a trinket before treatment. A little gift may well take his or her mind off the actual work being done. Tell a child there will be another one afterward—as a "thank-you" for his or her cooperation.

3. Question the child. Some examples can be "What is your favorite TV program?," "What is your favorite food?" and "If you could be anything in the world, what would you like to be when you grow up?"

4. If the child is cooperative, praise him or her to the skies. This type of emotional reinforcement goes a long way to making the child (and the adult patient, too) feel good. You can always say, if there is a grain of truth in it, "You're one of the doctor's *best* patients," or "You're one of the doctor's *favorite* patients."

5. Have a bulletin-board display of children's photos. Put the date on each photo. Children love to see themselves grow and change.

158

How to create a favorable office environment. It is the responsibility of the auxiliaries to make sure the office is a happy place. The colors used to decorate, the amount of lighting and the pictures hung on the walls all contribute.

We've seen offices filled with clowns, with mobiles, and very effectively, with posters filled with amusing sayings.

The office must always be absolutely spotless. A dirty office is a real turn-off. So is a dingy, poorly lighted one. Remember the waiting room and the business office are the places which make the first impression on the patient.

Tell people of the financial assistance you're helping them to get.
Many patients have dental coverage of one kind or another. It is definitely worthwhile to explain to the patients exactly how you are working on their behalf so that they are spared expense.

Whenever both husband and wife work, there is the possibility of coinsurance—to insure that the entire bill is paid. The office manager should check this out carefully, since it is possible to obtain thousands of dollars in benefits—to which the patient is entitled.

Offering discounts. The policy of offering discounts for cash payments has proven to be an effective practice builder. Of course you would set this policy with the doctor. We have used five percent of the figure with success. Along with this offer goes the assurance that the work is exactly the same as that done for the full price.

A "logo" for the office. Any type of theme or logo is appropriate. For example, you may suggest to the doctor one such as "Smile Center." This theme is excellent psychologically because the emphasis is a very pleasant one. You can then use a "logo" of a smile and place pictures of smiling faces throughout the office. You can even photograph your patients and use their pictures.

This has been carried as far as having the staff wear T-shirts with the logo, and actually distributing such T-shirts to patients.

Practice building

Another possible logo involves "Home Care," and still another is "Good Dental Health." The theme aspect may be carried throughout the office.

Put your doctor's name in front of your patients. The more often patients see the doctor's name, the more likely they are to come in for checkups, and the more likely they are to refer their family and friends to him or her.

Where can you have the doctor's name imprinted? Suggest toothbrushes, which are a logical choice, and hand mirrors.

Whenever you give a patient anything in writing, it must be on the office letterhead. This includes instructions for postoperative care, for example, or appointment cards.

The doctor may wish to distribute commercial materials, such as those available from the Dairy Council. Here, too, his or her name should appear on them.

Advertising. In some states advertising by dentists is relatively new, whereas in others it has been done for ages. The dental office manager can assist the doctor by finding the best places and methods for advertising. The following are possibilities: The Yellow Pages of the phone book, the local town or city newspaper, the TV guide for your area, local community newspapers, and "throwaways."

Newsletters. This type of publication can be sent to all of your doctor's patients—or to everyone in the community whose name appears on a voting list.

It should contain articles of general interest—such as the dangers of undetected high blood pressure—and also articles concerning your office, and the services offered. This type of "soft sell" may prove to be very effective. Furthermore, a newsletter may be sent as often as one chooses. It serves as a reminder of your doctor's office and services.

An 8½ x 11" sheet can be folded in thirds, with one portion containing the address; thereby eliminating the need for an envelope. Use a distinctive color that it will be associated with your office.

Announcements. Announcements are another reminder that may be sent to all present and former patients, thereby using your outdated files, and to an entire mailing list such as the voting list for your community.

The announcement may indicate new office hours, new services offered (e.g. that of a hygienist), new staff members, a new address or even a new orientation. (Dr. X announces the opening of the Smile Center.)

Sending greeting cards. Another aspect of personal attention is the sending of greeting cards. These may be for Christmas, for birthdays or other occasions, but they serve your purpose as they are reminders of your office. Humorous cards have been very well received by our patients.

Holding open house. Your doctor may wish to bring a volume of people into the office. This may be done by holding an "open house." Use the voting registration list to send invitations.

You must have some sort of interesting program to offer. "How to keep your teeth until the age of 100" might be one, or maybe "How to have a really dazzling smile." Whichever one you choose, have a definite program set up and we suggest you include refreshments. Make sure you have everything planned—including the flow of traffic through your office, and that the office is brightly lit, cheerful, decorated with fresh flowers and filled with people. When you send out your invitations, include an R.S.V.P., so that you will be able to intelligently plan for the number of guests you expect to come.

Telephone manners. Make sure the answering service you use is as pleasant and polite as you are. Answering services can be very impersonal—and deadly. Try to find one which answers on the first ring, and where the cheerful attitude of your office is carried through.

It goes without saying that patients who leave messages should receive a return call as soon as possible. New patients should be seen immediately if they are in pain. Otherwise they should be scheduled as soon as is convenient.

Your employer may prefer to use an answering machine. If so, be sure to leave a number that patients may call in an emergency.

Public speaking. Should your doctor care to speak, prepare a news release which includes a brief synopsis of the topic

Practice building, commercial devices

chosen. "New Happenings in Dentistry" is one possibility. Right now the process of bonding is receiving lots of attention. Circulate the news release, and you will probably find takers for your doctor's services. You may even be called to help him or her to prepare the speech. If so, make sure that the speech is warm and friendly.

Practice building, commercial devices.

Stickers. Youngsters love "stickers"—labels that they paste on their notebooks, their tote bags, their jackets— virtually everything. Attractive, inexpensive ones relating amusingly to dentistry are available from **Semantodoxtics, Inc**.

From the same firm may be purchased a variety of creative resources such as a *Children's Tooth Stool,* or a *Tooth Fairy Pillow* that lighten the tone of the office. Hardcovered, colorful, un- usual, handpainted solid-wood plaques with such messages as "Give your friends something to smile about. Tell them about our office," are an attractive way to get messages across, as are simpler messages such as "Thank you for the courtesy of Not Smoking."

It's fun to read the catalog. Send for it to **Semantodoxtics Inc.**, 3714 Indian School Road, PO Box 15668, Phoenix, AZ 85060.

Bumper stickers and cards. "I Love My Dentist" and a vari- ety of other creative stickers, buttons, umbrellas, recall cards, birthday cards and an ingenious "Thank you for helping us keep our practice blooming" card, which contains indoor seeds, soil and mailer are available, and appropriate gifts for patient as well.

Many such clever ideas are included in **Maxine's** catalog, 4830 Encino Avenue, Encino, CA 91316.

Shape up your smile, America! **Kerr/Syborn** has a program called *Shape Up Your Smile, America* which places great empha- sis on the esthetic aspect of dentistry. Their program consists of the following components:

1. A quarterly marketing newsletter that discusses how to mar- ket esthetic dentistry to your patients.

162

2. Patient information booklets such as "Let us improve your photo finish," and "Share your smile . . . Don't hide it!"
3. Technique folders.
4. A patient video tape.

For information, call 1-800-521-2854.

Motivational material for children's dentistry. A catalog is available from the American Society of Dentistry for Children with a variety of effective materials. For example, included is a certificate entititled "Official Dentist's Helper Award," and balloons with appropriate messages such as "Up, up and away with tooth decay." There is even a booklet on "Home Dental Care for the Infant." Write **American Society of Dentistry for Children,** 211 East Chicago Avenue, Suite 920, Chicago, IL 60611.

Newsletters. There are a number of newsletters available that offer practical advice. The information contained is geared to either the doctor or to his or her office manager.

One such newsletter is *Update and Practice Guidebook Reports* published by **Procom,** 5799 Tall Oaks Road, Madison, Wisconsin 53711.

Typical articles include: "Five Ways to Reduce Cancellations and No-Shows" and "How to Spot a Bad Check—in Advance!"

Precautionary measures. As a dental assistant, you are subject to a number of dangers which can be avoided without too much difficulty. For example, if you wear eyeglasses your eyes are protected from the debris which may result when the dental drill is being used. This is particularly true in four-handed dentistry. If, however, you do not wear glasses, it is suggested you do so. Safety glasses are a possibility, although you may feel that ordinary glasses, with "window pane" lenses are more attractive, and will serve the purpose.

You may want to wear a face mask while working on patients, particularly in the winter season, when upper respiratory ailments are transferred very readily. With the advent of the water-cooled drill, more and more bacteria are placed in the air in the immediate vicinity of the patient, and a mask is definitely indicated because of this. If your doctor does not wear one, you can certainly suggest it to him or her, since his or her health is also at stake.

Air pollution (*Mercury*, in particular) and radiation (*X-rays*) are discussed in other entries.

Preparing the operatory. It is important that the operatory and instruments be ready before the patient enters the room.

The following are duties of the dental assistant:

The chair should be adjusted to a position that facilitates the easiest entry, with bracket table and armrests out of the way.

A fresh saliva ejector and cup of water or mouthwash should be in place, as well as fresh bracket table cover and headrest cover.

All instruments should be readily accessible but out of sight of the patient.

Greet the patient and usher him or her into the chair. Make the patient as comfortable as possible.

The dental light and swinging bracket table should be positioned only after the patient is comfortable.

Bring the light and the bracket table to within reach of the dentist so that he or she will be able to adjust them. Try to avoid shining the dental light into a patient's eyes.

Most offices use disposable patient napkins, which are held in place by "Daisy chains." These are a pair of alligator clips held in place by a rope or chain. Slip the chain behind the patient's head and fasten the clip to the napkin on either side of the patient's shoulder.

The patient is now ready for the doctor to begin work.

Prescription requests over the phone. No staff member except the doctor can authorize prescriptions. Therefore, if a patient or a pharmacist telephones, the doctor must take this call, and make all the necessary arrangements.

For controlled substances, no prescription can be given over the telephone. The patient must come into the office and see the doctor to obtain a prescription for this type of medication.

Preventive dentistry. In many dental offices it is the role of the dental assistant to teach effective methods of preventive dentistry to the patients.

It is essential that the program be designed with your employer's ideas and input. One of the best ways to do this is by sitting down together and working out a basic plan—which should then be varied to suit the needs of the individual patient.

Your basic plan would probably include the following items:

Motivation. This would include information as to why a patient needs to care for his or her dental health. It should discuss what can be achieved by a person who will conscientiously follow a preventive program and may (or may not) include what can happen if he or she does not follow such a program.

The use of audio-visual material of all types is very valuable in motivating patients in this regard.

Setting goals. Taking into consideration the patient's personality and previous behavior, goals should be set up. These goals must be realistic. If a patient has not been conscientious up to this time, one cannot expect him or her to brush (or anything else) after every meal. It is far more effective to try to get this patient to brush once a day.

Specific procedures to be followed must be taught. These should first be demonstrated and then the patient should perform them. It is the dental assistant's function to see to it that they are performed correctly. This includes methods for brushing, flossing, tipping, etc. Since this step is the very basis for the preventive program, it must be done with extreme care and attention to detail.

Follow-up. Since a goal has been established, it is possible to do part of the follow-up by telephone. The dental assistant may call the patient, asking if he or she is being conscientious in carrying out this program.

165

Professional literature for patients

The second part of the follow-up is by a return visit by the patient. When dealing with children, particularly, but with adults as well, patience and pleasantness are the key words. Everyone involved in dentistry is aware of the fact that there are some people who will not carry out a program of preventive dentistry. However, there are those that will. The dental assistant's role as a teacher here is to convert those who are resistant and encourage and support those who are already carrying out the program.

Professional literature for patients. While seated in your waiting room, patients (and people waiting for them) usually seek something to read. This is an excellent time to provide them with professional literature. Most patients need to be educated in terms of dental health, and this is an opportune time to begin this. It is also a good time to review the dental services available to them. All materials should be put in a prominent place, and kept neat, clean and current. Literature to take home is an excellent means of getting the message across.

There are a number of sources of material.

Your doctor may choose to write his own text, which can be duplicated easily. This may be in the form of "Fact Sheets," (call them "Smile Sheets" if you like) or newsletters. If he or she writes on them, it is a good idea to have them reflect his or her personal concern by writing directly to the patient, and not a cold, scientific treatise. A staff member, if talented, might do the writing if the doctor so decides.

Commercial materials are available from many companies, and while they are advertisements, they can still be valuable in giving patients information.

The **American Dental Association, Bureau of Health, Education and Audio-visual Services,** 211 East Chicago Avenue, Chicago, IL 60611 has a variety of excellent material, available at low cost.

Check with the following: **The National Dairy Council,** 6300 North River Road, Rosemont, IL 60018; **The American Cancer Society,** 4 West 35th Street, New York, NY 10001; **The Metropolitan Life Insurance Company, Health and Safety Education Division,** 1 Madison Avenue, New York, NY 10010.

People love to get "freebies," and so any material you offer will probably be taken home and, hopefully be read. They certainly can do no harm. Have a stamp for placing the name, address and telephone number of your practice somewhere on the literature.

Progress reports from patients.   Sometimes the dentist will ask patients to "let me know how you are getting along." For example, he might ask after oral surgery. When patients call in to report good progress, make a written record of the call and submit it to the doctor.

Should a patient wish to speak to the doctor, tell the patient you will have the doctor call as soon as he or she is finished seeing the present patient. Only in the case of an emergency should the call be put through.

See *Telephone Call Report* for a form which may be used.

Public relations.   All members of the staff of any business or organization are involved in public relations, which is the image or impression patients and the general public get of that business or organization. In this case it is the image of your doctor and his or her office staff.

To begin with, you should respect the doctor and the patients, and treat everyone in that way. Your behavior should be warm but professional, interested but never nosy.

You will often be called upon for explanations which can clear the air and dispel doubts in the patient's minds. You will also be called upon to give the patients emotional support. Your warmth and understanding will help patients and your doctor as well.

Never, ever give nasty or rude responses to anyone. Be kind and courteous to every patient. The growth and health of a dental practice depends as much upon the patient's image of it as upon the skill of the doctor. This point cannot be overemphasized.

Being gentle and pleasant may be difficult when you're having a terribly busy day—but the way you treat patients can make a big difference in the success of the practice.

167

Ask your doctor questions, when necessary. If there is something you need to know don't hesitate to ask for the information you want. Find out the way the doctor wants you to do things, and do them that way.

If you think you may know a better way, then, when he or she has time, discuss it—but if the doctor still wishes them done his or her way, don't argue about it.

When you make a mistake, do not try to give a lengthy explanation. Merely admit it, learn what is expected of you and do it. Long explanations often make the person more irritated.

If, at the end of a busy day, your doctor is not as pleasant as normally, remember there is a great deal of tension and anxiety connected with his or her work. Be understanding of this.

Never, ever, under any circumstances should you argue with your employer in the presence of a patient. Remember—the doctor is the boss! Never criticize him or her, or even complain. Present, as part of your public relations program, a pleasant, confident united office, with all personnel working for the good of the patient.

Your telephone communication is important, too; (see *Telephone*) as is your written communication. Always, for example, answer the telephone as instructed. Use the doctor's stationery even when writing a short memo.

Sending Christmas cards is one aspect of public relations which should be considered. Most patients appreciate being remembered and acknowledged, particularly at that time of the year.

Pulling files.   Patient files should be pulled from the day sheet list that is prepared by the office manager. This job may be delegated to either the office manager or the dental assistant. Be sure to always leave a card or marker in place of the file; this minimizes refiling time.

It is best to pull the following day's charts before leaving the office the evening before.

The assistant should look the chart over to familiarize herself with the procedure scheduled for that visit; it can save valuable time by being able to simply tell the doctor the procedure to be done and what tooth or quadrant should be anesthetized.

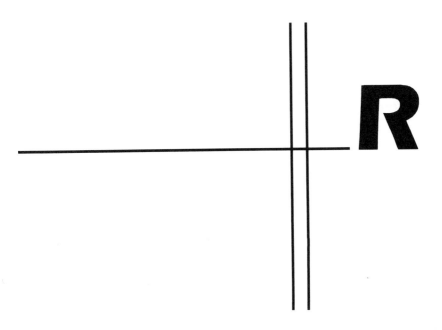

Recalls. An efficient recall system is important, and relatively simple to maintain.

Postcards or letters should be printed with words to the effect:

Office logo

Doctor's name
Address
Telephone number

Dear _____,
A period of six months has elapsed since your last appointment. Because your dental health requires a semiannual checkup, we are making an appointment for your visit on
_____ at A.M./P.M.

If this time is inconvenient, please telephone us to reschedule it.

We know you are concerned with your dental health, and that you realize the importance of this checkup. We look forward to seeing you.

Sincerely yours,
Jane Doe, Office Manager

Reference bookshelf

You will have filled out these postcards or letters during the patient's previous appointment, after treatment had been completed. Write the date into the doctor's or the hygienist's appointment book, along with the patient's telephone number.

Then place the card or letter in a file which has each month divided into halves. When that month is reached, all the office manager need do is mail the cards or letters two to three weeks in advance of the appointment.

The next step consists of calling the patient one week before the date of the appointment to confirm. Confirmation is absolutely essential.

If there are patients the doctor does not wish to have recalled, he or she must give this information to the office manager before the postcard or letter is filled out—or, if it has already been done, the card may be removed from the file.

Since there is often dental work that must be redone because it has outlived its usefulness, or because new techniques are available, "recalls" provide a significant source of income for the office.

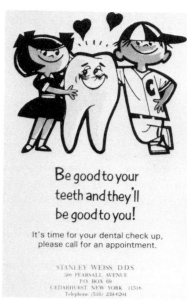
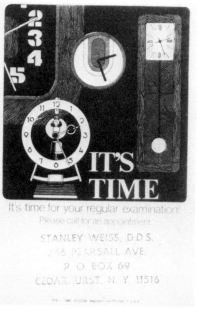

Reference bookshelf.   You should have a collection of books to help you. These books will save you precious time and often money. Here are some you will probably find useful to have close to your desk.

170

Telephone directories.   Both yellow and white pages. If you have not already discovered just how valuable having these books easily available is, you will be amazed that you never thought of this before.

Be sure to obtain all of the directories that are published for your area. This would include all of the suburbs as well as the major city.

If you must deal frequently with other cities, telephone the business office of the telephone company in those cities and request copies of the phonebook.

If you use certain sections of the yellow pages, turn down the upper corner and place a staple through the triangle formed. This will serve as a marker, making use of the book quicker and easier.

When you discover a number in the book has been changed, change it in the directory as well.

A dictionary.   For spelling and pronunciation a dictionary is very valuable. You need a desk-sized book rather than a library-type volume.

A ZIP code book.   This book helps you to properly address your mail, without wasting time calling the post office to find out what a particular ZIP code should be.

Do not send out mail without a ZIP code, because it may be returned to you, thereby wasting valuable time. See *ZIP code.*

Referral, thank-you.   It is good manners, and good business, to thank patients when they refer their friends to your office. There are many ways that you can do this. One is by a personal letter, such as the one that follows:

Dear Mrs. X,

Thank you for referring ———————————————— to me for dental treatment. You may be sure that I will do my utmost for ————————, and I want you to know I appreciate your confidence in me.

With warmest wishes.

Sincerely,

Dr. James Brown

This letter should be signed by the doctor, personally.

Referral

Your employer may decide to enlarge upon this. Successful practitioners have sent small gifts—a single rose, for example, or a scarf. Again, the doctor's personal signature is important.

If a patient has referred a number of patients, the gift should be more impressive. A plant, a bouquet of flowers or a book are possibilities, with a warm personal note. The following is an e xample of such a note.

Dear Mrs. X,

Over the years my practice has grown because of patients like yourself who have been appreciative of my work, and kind enough to recommend me to others.

I have always given everyone the best dental care possible and, of course, will continue to do so in the future. However, it is people like you who lift my spirits, and for this and your belief in me I am most grateful.

Sincerely,

Dr. James Brown

Reminder system. Use a desk calendar or card file for this purpose. Do not be tempted to use the appointment book.

Write in, as far as you can, all of the special dates you know of in advance. You may find it useful to indicate school holidays, if your doctor sees young people frequently. Record all holidays when the office is closed.

When dates such as meeting notices are received in the mail, note them on the desk calendar.

The index-card file is used in the same manner. A commercially prepared one may be purchased, with a card for each date, and tabs for each month.

Items of both personal and business nature should be listed. These would include the following:

Birthdays of all family members—the immediate family, those suggested by the doctor and others you feel are important.

Anniversaries

Meetings

172

Payment dates for mortgages, loans, car payments, insurance premiums and interest on notes.

License renewals for driving and auto registration.

Tax dates—such as April 1 rather than April 15, when the Federal Income Tax return is due. Also remember state and city taxes.

Special Entries:

Patient birthdates
Christmas cards

This reminder system should be checked one week in advance, so that necessary action may be taken before the due date.

Follow-up file. A tickler file can help you remember things which must be followed up. Keep a separate file for this purpose.

Write up an index card for each item which needs further action. Place the date on which the follow-up should be done, and file it under that date.

Check this file daily. Items entered might include:

Send out progress report on Mary Smith to Dr. Jones.

Lab reports due back on Jones, Roger and Brown.

Make reservations for dinner for five at Blue Tree Lodge.

Call patients who have appointments for the following day (list of patients).

Send out thank-you for referral from Dr. Brown.

Retraction and suction. As previously stated, the prime responsibility of the dental assistant is to aid the dentist at the chair. For any procedure requiring the use of a high-speed handpiece, the lips, cheeks, and tongue must be protected, and the water spray continuously evacuated from the mouth.

The instrument most commonly used for this protection is a mouth mirror. Initially, the dentist may direct you as to where to place the mirror; soon you will become adept at this. Supplemental retraction may be accomplished with cotton rolls, tissue retractors or the rubber dam.

The most common evacuation device is the saliva ejector. This is usually a plastic tube that connects to a hose running up the side of the dental unit that has the cuspidor on it. The tube is flexible and can be bent to fit, but avoid bending it over on itself into a "U." Strength of suction is controlled by a valve. This type of suction device functions best for picking up water spray; for surgical procedures that involve bleeding, a high-speed evacuator may be used. This may be found adjacent to the other hose, or in a portable unit. These ejectors are larger in bore, and may have a right-angle bend and beveled-bore tips, or be straight with bevelled ends. These devices evacuate at a much greater rate, and are therefore more dangerous. They should be used sparingly and with care; they should never be left in the patient's mouth as they can pinch the tissues severely.

The most common method of readying the patient for a procedure is to place the saliva ejector first, then the mirror for retraction, and finally the drill and mirror if the dentist is using one.

Be aware that it is common for patients to constantly want to sit up and spit in the cuspidor. This is delaying behavior that can drive a dentist to distraction. Effective use of a saliva ejector can prevent this and increase productivity.

You will find that this entire procedure will soon become automatic and easy.

Routines, importance of.   Routines make the work of each person easier. A routine is a procedure which is followed on a daily basis. When activities have become "routinized," they require relatively little concentration, and therefore go quickly and almost effortlessly.

For example, routines should be developed for the opening of the office. Such things as pulling up shades, turning off alarm systems, putting on lights and emptying waste baskets are just some of the items that comprise the office-opening routine. All of these procedures should be listed in an Office Manual so that if the staff member who normally performs these activities is absent, another may take her place.

Make routines as simple as possible. For example, when emptying wastebaskets, place the contents in disposable plastic

174

bags, rather than in another container. Have these bags placed where they are easily accessible.

Once a routine has been perfected and memorized, all the details will be taken care of, thus insuring a smoothly running office.

Rubber dam. The rubber dam is a device employed to increase the visibility of the operating field, to minimize contamination by saliva and isolate the tooth or teeth being worked on. While a rubber dam is especially valuable in endodontics (because in addition to the other reasons, it prevents accidental swallowing of an instrument), some dentists employ it regularly when doing operative procedures as well. It may be part of your job to assist the doctor in readying and placing the dam.

The rubber dam itself is a sheet of latex rubber, approximately 5x5", in which holes are punched to correspond to the area being isolated. The rubber dam punch is used to make these holes. It is an instrument that resembles a forceps, with a pointed end on one side and a rotating disc with various-sized holes opposite it. The largest holes are punched for molars and the smallest for anterior teeth. If available, a stamp can be applied to the rubber dam itself with a formula corresponding to the dentition. You then punch holes for whatever teeth are being isolated. In time, you will not need the stamp.

Once in place, the dam is fixed by clamping a metal clamp onto a tooth. There are a variety of such clamps available, either for isolating a single tooth that will be worked on, or those adjacent to it. A frame is then placed around the patient's face to support the rubber.

There are two methods of rubber dam placement. In one, the dam is punched and placed over the teeth, then clamped and stretched over the frame. In the other, the entire assembly (frame, dam and clamp) is assembled outside the mouth and placed as one unit. A forceps is used to engage the holes in the wings of the clamp; the clamp is then separated to provide space to fit over the tooth and locked by moving the metal ring down the forcep until it locks in place. The clamp is applied at the gingival margin of the tooth and the locking mechanism released. Finally, warm air and a plastic instrument is used to tuck the edges of the rubber dam firmly around the tooth to seal out saliva. Dental floss may be used to force the dam through the contact area if necessary.

It is good practice to either vaseline the lips and cheek before placement of the rubber dam, or use a special napkin around the mouth before placing the dam.

It is often easier to place the saliva ejector before applying the dam.

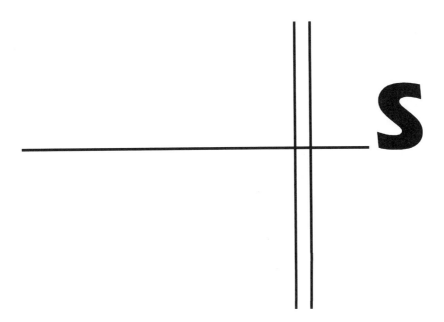

Safety in the office.   Dentists, like other citizens, are responsible for their offices and may be sued by persons injured on the premises. It is the responsibility of the office personnel to make those areas as safe as possible.

1. Make sure all doors open and close easily.
2. Use a nonslip floor polish, and make sure that the floors are not slippery after washing or waxing.
3. Be sure all equipment is clean and free of germs.
4. Be sure all equipment is in good operating order.
5. Be sure no person unable to care for himself or herself is left alone. This rule applies to the elderly, the ill and the very young, in the treatment room or the bathroom.
6. Help any patient who is unable to walk.
7. Do not allow patients to open or close windows.
8. Supply ashtrays if smoking is permitted in your office.
9. Make sure all pathways within the office are unobstructed.
10. Make sure the office is well lit.

The doctor carries accident-liability insurance policies. However, it is up to office manager to make sure premiums are paid so that the coverage is in effect.

Setting the tone of the office.   Office Managers set the tone of the dental office because they are the first employees to make contact with a patient.

Patients are frequently worried and tense when they enter the office. You should be warm, cordial and not too immersed in your own work to fail to be available to talk to for at least a few minutes. In that time you should attempt to put the patient at ease by inquiring about the patient's well-being, his or her family, the state of the weather, current events or just making small talk. This act of putting the patient at ease, if successful, is an excellent practice builder, and also makes the doctor's task easier.

Your dealings with the patient can literally make you a tremendous asset, or a liability, to your employer.

In dealing with patients you should never discuss anything regarding one patient with another. If a person is "fishing" to find out if Mrs. X is one of the doctor's patients, a response such as "Oh, do you know Mrs. X?" is adequate. Even if she isn't, the response will do.

You should not give dental advice. but should check with the doctor at all times. Giving the wrong advice could harm the patient, and possibly the doctor, as well. When asked a specific question, you should respond by saying, "I'll check with the doctor."

All patients should be treated the same way, regardless of their financial status. Your attitude should be one of sincere interest in each and every patient.

If the doctor is "running late," and not on time for his appointments, explain the delay. Patients often build up "a head of steam" while waiting. If the delay is unavoidable, explain it and apologize, saying with a smile, "The doctor really cannot help keeping you waiting. Thank you so much for your patience."

Shopper's, how to handle.   You undoubtedly receive phone calls from patients who are "shopping," and who want you to quote fees over the phone. Whether you do or do not will depend on your employer's policy, so discuss this in full detail.

Before deciding whether you should give the caller the exact information, your employer should know that a fee quoted is often considered to be a legal contract. Since each patient has different needs, it is unwise to set fees by telephone.

Remember, this potential patient gets his or her first impression from your reaction over the telephone. You can favorably impress him or her by having a smile in your voice. On the other hand, if you are annoyed, that, too, will come across. So, first, thank the patient for telephoning your office.

Instead of giving figures, discuss with the shopper (who we'll call "her") the concept that her health is at stake, and that since she is an individual with unique needs, it is impossible for any conscientious dental assistant to quote fees over the telephone that would be fair to both the patient and the dentist. Point out the fact that in your office she will receive the best possible care, and that the fees charged are comparable with those charged by other dentists in the area.

Ask if the patient is in pain, and assure her that your employer will take care of the offending tooth, if she so desires, at the earliest opportunity.

Whatever the patient's reaction, be sure to avoid any unpleasantness; it is important to leave her with a favorable impression of your office. She will then remain a potential patient.

As you gain experience, you will become adept at categorizing the patient's complaints. A caller who complains of a "toothache" in all likelihood will need a sedative temporary filling or deep gingival scaling—procedures that do not require excessive time. It is a big plus to tell the caller she can be seen quickly.

Shorthand.   As office manager, if you do not know shorthand, you would benefit from learning it. Courses offering techniques that use letters rather than symbols, such as *Speedwriting,* are generally mastered in a shorter period of time.

If you do not care to learn a system, develop your own shorthand. To develop your own system, you will have to observe your written work and study it carefully. Determine which words are used frequently, and develop your own symbols for them. Other people will not be able to transcribe your notes, but since this is rarely done anyway, it will not present a problem.

For example, the capital letter "D" may be used instead of the word "Dear" in writing a letter. "VTY" may be "Very truly Yours." Do the same thing for dental terms.

If you develop your own terms, however, based on your own needs, you will probably find them more useful than standard forms.

"Short-notice" patients.   Keep a listing of patients who can come in on short notice. You can obtain this by asking patients, when they are making appointments, if they are available to come in earlier if a change in scheduling should occur. Place their names and phone numbers where they are readily available. Ask them which days of the week and what times of the day they are available, and how long it takes them to get to your office.

By referring to this information you are able to fill in when cancellations occur, and avoid the waste of valuable time.

Since this is definitely an accommodation on the part of the patients, make sure to verbally indicate your appreciation that they are willing to change their plans.

Women who do not work outside the home and senior citizens will probably form the major portion of your "short-notice" list. Self-employed people, too, are good prospects. The more patients you locate who are available, the easier your task of filling cancelled time will be.

Slander and irresponsible remarks.   Dental auxiliaries are sometimes placed in a position where it is possible to "say the wrong thing." It is essential one be highly circumspect and avoid careless or unthinking remarks.

Here are some examples of what *not* to say:

"I can't understand why Dr. X did this work. You probably didn't need it."

"You should be taking _____ (some form of medication). It will help you a lot. It helped my brother-in-law."

"Dr. X is always late. You'll have to get used to that!"

"Dr. Z did that to you? He should be sued."

It is incredible, but these remarks have actually been made.

It is not your job to determine the condition of the patient, prescribe medication or denigrate any other professional.

It is your job to be supportive of all patients, without commenting on anything other than superficial things. This does not imply that you are undeservedly protecting or covering up anything done by other doctors. Rather, it is a recognition that you do not have all the available information, and so cannot knowledgeably comment on things that occurred away from your office.

Smoking policy. The doctor is the person who will establish the policy for smoking or nonsmoking in his or her office. However, since smoking is detrimental not only to the health of the smoker but to nonsmokers as well, it is valuable to establish certain rules regarding it.

The dental office is a health care facility, and as such should be kept as free of air pollution as possible. Therefore, a room or lounge may be set aside to accommodate staff members who smoke. Signs should be placed in the waiting room stating "Thank you for not smoking. Smoking is dangerous to your health."

If you are a smoker, try to wean yourself. It is you, personally, who will benefit more than anyone else. You are surely aware of your increased vulnerability to lung cancer and heart disease.

Should you be in a position to hire personnel, you can consider employing only nonsmokers. If a person is a heavy smoker, it is necessary to consider carefully whether or not you want her working in your office. The doctor who does not smoke may not want a smoker in his employ.

Stain removal. It is important to be able to remove stains and discolorations which are bound to occur in any office. Uniforms, for example, because they are usually solid color, should be kept as spot-free as possible.

State abbreviations

Some of the most frequent stains and the means to remove them follow:

Blood: Soak in cold water, as soon as possible. Use a detergent. Rub the stain against another part of the fabric. If the stain does not come out entirely, test the fabric with hydrogen peroxide. If it doesn't injure the fabric, use it on the stain. Avoid warm or hot water.

Coffee: Use warm water plus Wisk or a similar detergent.

Ballpoint pen ink: Cover stain with petroleum jelly. Remove grease with a grease solvent. Repeat until stain comes out.

Chewing gum: Apply ice to the gum. Scrape off with a dull knife, being careful not to damage the fabric. Repeat until no more gum comes off. Use a grease solvent on remainder.

State abbreviations. The post office has requested the use of the following state abbreviations because of the electronic sorting of mail:

Alabama	AL	Montana	MT
Alaska	AK	Nebraska	NE
Arizona	AZ	Nevada	NV
Arkansas	AR	New Hampshire	NH
California	CA	New Jersey	NJ
Colorado	CO	New Mexico	NM
Connecticut	CT	New York	NY
Delaware	DE	North Carolina	NC
District of Columbia	DC	North Dakota	ND
Florida	FL	Ohio	OH
Georgia	GA	Oklahoma	OK
Hawaii	HI	Oregon	OR
Idaho	ID	Pennsylvania	PA
Illinois	IL	Puerto Rico	PR
Indiana	IN	Rhode Island	RI
Iowa	IA	South Carolina	SC
Kansas	KS	South Dakota	SD

Kentucky	KY	Tennessee	TN
Louisiana	LA	Texas	TX
Maine	ME	Utah	UT
Maryland	MD	Vermont	VT
Massachusetts	MA	Virginia	VA
Michigan	MI	Virgin Islands	VI
Minnesota	MN	Washington	WA
Mississippi	MS	West Virginia	WV
Missouri	MO	Wisconsin	WI
		Wyoming	WY

Steam sterilization of instruments. Moist heat, in the form of steam, is the most effective means of sterilization. The autoclave is used for this purpose; the word evolving from "auto" meaning "self," and "clave" meaning "closing." The autoclave is kept tightly closed because the pressure of the steam forces it to be so. It must be used by following the instructions to the letter. If the temperature is not exactly what it should be, the material placed in it may not be sterilized, or may be destroyed by superheating.

Study the instruction booklet carefully. It will teach you exactly how to clean and care for the apparatus. If you do not have a copy of this booklet, write to the manufacturer for one.

The autoclave is used for the sterilization of instruments *after* they have been washed clean. To wash them, first soak the instruments in warm water to which a detergent such as *Haemosole* or *Edisonite* has been added.

Next scrub with a stiff hand brush, making sure all particles, however small, have been removed. Tissue and blood may tend to remain unless scrubbed off. Rinse with boiling water and dry.

When the instruments are clean, place on a wire-mesh or perforated-bottom tray in the autoclave and steam under pressure at a temperature of 250 degrees Fahrenheit (121 degrees Centigrade) for a minimum of fifteen minutes, or 270 degrees Fahrenheit (132 degrees Centigrade) for a minimum of seven minutes. Be sure to place a layer of muslin or paper towel in the bottom of the tray.

Sterile conditions

All instruments should be placed on the tray open or un-locked, and not touching each other. Cover the instruments with a layer of muslin.

After the period of steaming is over, allow the instruments to remain in the sterilizer for 15 minutes with the door open one-quarter inch to insure thorough drying.

Note: Sharp-edged instruments are injured by heat, and should be sterilized by placing in 70 percent alcohol for ten to twenty minutes. Another method is to place in boiling water, and boil for ten minutes. Remove at once with sterile forceps, and while still hot, shake off excess water and place in sterile container.

Surgical instruments are often cleaned, wrapped in paper, then placed in individual bags, with the identification of the in-strument pencilled on the bag. A stripe on the bag turns color after autoclaving, and is a "fail-safe" way of insuring sterility. The bag is stapled or glued closed, and kept that way until opened. The bag should be dated before being placed in the ap-propriate drawer.

Dry-heat sterilization is accomplished in a dry-heat oven, and is beneficial for sterilization of items that cannot be auto-claved. The range of heat produced in the oven can vary from 100 to 200 degrees Centigrade. The most frequent technique uses overnight sterilization at 121 degrees Centigrade and must be done for at least six hours.

Endodontic instruments such as files, reamers and broaches are also sterilized by use of a glass bead sterilizer, which as its name implies, employs heated beads of glass in a small container. Instruments are placed in the hot beads for ap-proximately five seconds, with the plastic handles of the instru-ments left in the air. Prolonged immersion of the metal results in increasing weakness, with the possibility of them breaking in the root canal greatly increased.

Sterile conditions. It is extremely necessary that you observe sterile conditions constantly.

Between patients, equipment in the operatory which has been splattered should be wiped with a disinfectant, such as iodine or 70 percent isopropyl alcohol.

184

If you touch anything which might have bacteria on it, your hands should be washed, again, even though you've just washed them. This is true any time you leave the operatory, in the presence of the patient.

Should you cut yourself, or have any open wound, it must be kept covered by wearing gloves. This is for your protection, and is very necessary.

Sterilization. "Sterile" means absolutely free of all bacteria or other living organisms, and "sterilization" is the process whereby these organisms are killed. Since bacteria or germs often cause infection or disease, it is essential that any instrument be sterilized before the doctor touches the patient with it.

It is only since the late nineteenth century that sterilization has been used. Joseph Lister is generally credited with having introduced the concept into surgery.

Different methods are used for different materials. Some of the essentials used in the doctor's office are available already sterilized and packaged so that resterilization is unnecessary. These include bandages, gloves, gauze, syringes and needles, oral-surgery instruments and suturing materials.

Sterilization differs from disinfection and germicide. Disinfectants usually kill disease-producing bacteria, but do not kill those which form spores. Disinfectants include certain chemicals, boiling water, flowing steam and ultraviolet radiation. A disinfectant should never be used on the body of any person.

Germicides kill bacteria. As with disinfectants, they do not generally kill spores. Germicides may be applied to parts of the human body, as well as to objects. Other names by which germicides may be called include bacteriocides and fungicides.

Antiseptic comes from the terms "anti" meaning against and "sepsis" meaning disease. Antiseptics either kill bacteria or cause them to become harmless, and are made to be used on living tissues. See *Steam sterilization.*

Stocking the office. Part of your duties in the office may involve maintaining and stocking the supplies used on a daily basis. This is vital, for running out of an item may cause enormous problems for you and your employer.

185

The easiest way to insure that this never happens is by keeping track of items as they are taken from storage. You should compile a master list of all supplies stocked in the office, what quantity of an item is on hand, what has been removed and when and where that item may be ordered.

You can start a master list by hand, or develop one from a catalog or manual. It should be kept close to the supplies themselves, and once a week you should check to see what materials must be ordered.

It is wise to plan to stock enough material to last at least two months. For materials that have a limited shelf life, check the expiration date that is printed on the box, and always use the older material (that is, those with the earliest expiration dates) before the newer.

Stress, how to handle your.   Your work, by its very nature, involves a good deal of stress, and it is important that you learn how to handle it so that it does not do you any harm physically or mentally.

Stress itself is not harmful, but is rather a normal part of life. Our bodies display what has been termed the "fight or flight" response, which is the name given to quickened pulse and breathing, release of adrenalin, release of blood sugar and changed muscle tone when the organism is threatened. One may also show changes in our digestion, in our circulating hormones, in our blood and possibly in our brain chemistry. These changes may be in response to such situations in the office as an overload of patients, patient complaints, equipment breakdowns, extra emergencies—or a variety of other reasons. Fear, anger, anxiety, frustration and guilt can all cause stress. Of course, events in one's personal life—such as the illness or death of a loved one, separation or divorce can cause stress—but so can happy events such as a wedding, becoming a parent or moving into a new residence.

Stress may manifest itself in different ways. Migraine or other types of headaches, backaches, shoulder pains or digestive disturbances may all be stress related, and may significantly effect the performance of the office as well as the quality of your life outside the office.

What can you do to minimize unnecessary stress? There are a number of steps you can take. First of all, by being prepared, you can avoid many potentially stressful situations. As we have mentioned in other entries, use of a tray system and learning to anticipate your doctor's needs in advance will make chairside assisting considerably less stressful, and make your employer more appreciative of your efforts.

Learn to anticipate and do as many things in advance as you possibly can. (We know of one dentist whose Christmas cards are addressed during the summer when his practice slows down a bit, rather than later on when the office is very busy.) This applies to all facets of the practice, such as emergency patients, ordering of materials and supplies, maintenance of equipment, preparing for inclement weather or any of the daily issues that may come up. As we have mentioned, the more routine your work is, the less investment in time and worry is necessary.

Detach yourself from situations where there is a little you can do to resolve them. Learn not to take these situations personally. If a patient complains, use active listening and speak softly to diffuse their anxiety. Often, they may be angry at pain they are experiencing, not at you or the doctor. In many cases, the best response you can give is to not give one at all, but to nod and look sympathetic. Try not to let things get you down. There is no one on earth who does not have problems of one sort or another. Remembering this can help you avoid stress.

Try not to allow yourself to become depressed. The effects of stress are cumulative, and while you may not be able to recognize the symptoms of an approaching depression, remember that depression is a physical illness that may be thought of as a lower level of electrical energy in your brain. Because of the stressful nature of working in a dental office, you should work to develop strategies to diffuse stress. We find physical activities, such as getting out of the office on your lunch hour and walking, or going shopping or lunching with friends, can be a big help in this regard. Mini-vacations, such as long weekends, or even two days, are useful because they help break the routine. (One highly successful dentist established a system of having a three-day weekend once a month—to alleviate his own pressure, as well as that of his staff.) You might suggest this to your employer.

Most dental offices have music, and that, too, will help avoid stress, providing the music is soothing.

Should you feel you are very stressed, or depressed, and need help, see your physician. It is possible that you may require medication to see you through your day's work, although this is rare. If you feel the necessity however, it may be worth checking out.

Sugar, damage done by. In educating patients, the role played by sugar is extremely important, and they need to understand it.

In what way does the eating of sugar affect the teeth? It has been shown by research that the amount of plaque (which are actually colonies of bacteria growing in the mouth) accumulates faster in the presence of sugar (sucrose). Since plaque is the cause of dental caries, by cutting down on sugar there will consequently be less tooth decay.

A completely carbohydrate-free or even a sucrose-free diet is not practical, but diminishing the amount of sugar can produce good results in terms of dental health.

It is interesting to note the fact that plaque does develop, even when no carbohydrates are present in the diet—but the quantity of bacteria is altered.

Supplies, ordering and storing. To keep the dental office well stocked, a complete inventory should be taken at least once a year. (See *Inventory*.) This is usually done by the dental assistant.

Once an inventory is done, a copy should be kept available, and when the supply of an item is running low, a new supply should be ordered. Never allow the supply of an item to run so low that you can possibly run out of it.

Try to avoid ordering small amounts of items. You waste your time and energy. Order sufficient quantities to cover your needs for a period of six months to one year.

Shop for a good price—particularly when you are buying in quantity. However, do not overorder. (A good criteria is to estimate the quantity of the item you use in six months, and order that amount.)

When a sample of a new product is offered, try it out—but do not be too quick to order it unless you find it superior to the product you have been using.

When an order is received take the time to carefully check it to make sure you are receiving the quantity of the item for which you are being billed. Do not sign a receipt for any order until you have checked it carefully.

Store your supplies so that you know where they are, and can get to them easily. This is best done by designating a place for each item.

When storing materials that deteriorate, such as letterheads, keep them in closed packages. Label such packages so there is no need to open them to determine the contents.

Of course your doctor may want to add other items to this listing, or omit some of those listed. It is advisable to check this with him or her once or twice a year.

You may find you can obtain a listing of this type of inventory from certain medical supply houses. Be sure, however, that you are free to order any item you wish, and not just those products that firm sells.

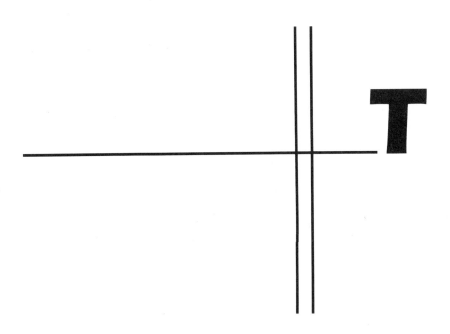

Teacher Education Programs for Dental Assistants. Dental Assistants interested in teaching can find the course of study necessary offered by the University of North Carolina at College Hill. The undergraduate curriculum leading to a B.S. degree includes courses in liberal arts, basic and dental sciences, education and dentally related education. There are graduate programs offered as well, leading to a Master of Science degree. These include a required core and two areas of concentration from Dental Auxiliary Utilization, Dental Radiology, Oral Pathology, Biologic Sciences, Clinical Laboratory Education and Education. There is a one semester internship required for both undergraduate and graduate programs. For information contact the **Dental Auxiliary Teacher Education,** University of North Carolina School of Dentistry, 328A Brauer Hall, Chapel Hill, N.C. 27514.

Graduate training is offered at Boston University's Goldman School of Graduate Dentistry. A nine-month program leading to a Master of Science degree includes dental health management, dental education and research with options for concentration in public health and nutrition. This program has been in existence for years, and prepares graduates for positions in dental education (in colleges and universities), clinical administration, government and private industry. For information: Registrar, Boston University Goldman School of Graduate Dentistry, 100 East Newton Street, Boston, Ma. 02118. Applicants should be certified dental assistants, and have a Bachelor's Degree, or its equivalent.

Teamwork. *Synergy* is a term that describes a relationship that is worth more than the sum of its parts, and is a good way to view a dental practice. In the same way that the routinizing of everyday tasks simplifies their performance, the interaction of a trained, motivated staff produces an effect of enhancing the practice, thus benefiting patient and staff alike. An efficiently run practice, based on a clear understanding by staff members of their respective duties is virtually guaranteed to be successful.

In the same way as the doctor is ultimately responsible for the care of the patients, much of the tone and feeling of the practice will be set by him or her. Find out how the doctor relates to his patients by observing his behavior with them. If he or she is outgoing and discusses his family with the patients, you may do the same. Consider your employer as a team leader and never hesitate to discuss problems or anything pertinent with him or her.

Make an effort to be constantly looking for ways to improve the office by easing the load of someone else and increasing your own efficiency. If you feel that there are problems that must be discussed among the staff, tell your employer, and suggest having a scheduled staff meeting on a regular basis to address these issues.

You will find that many problems arise over the responsibility of staff members to perform various tasks—again, the more specific your office manual is in terms of who takes the responsibility for a task, the less problems you will have.

Our culture places a special emphasis on facial looks and the importance of healthy teeth; as you spend more time in your office, you will undoubtlessly encounter people who show profound personality changes following restoration of their mouths. This should be as rewarding to you as it is to the dentist—you will find, as time goes by, that pride in a job well done is an important aspect of dentistry that is as rewarding as your paycheck, and a true source of satisfaction to all.

Telephone call report. Use the following form:

TELEPHONE CALL REPORT

Date _____

Patient's name _____

Purpose of call _____

_____

_____

_____

_____

_____

_____

_____

Action Taken:
    Appointment Made (Date) _____

    Message Delivered _____

    Letter Sent _____

Message Taken by: _____

Telephone information. The first section of your "white pages" telephone directory contains a great deal of information of value to the dental secretary. It is well worth the time required to review and familiarize yourself with it.

The following is a very brief summary:

1. A table of contents
2. Business contacts with the telephone company including telephone installation and bill payments

3. Services and Equipment
4. Office codes
5. Calling locally
6. Calling long distance—including rates, area codes and types of long-distance calls
7. Message-unit table
8. Other relevant information

You will find information regarding directory assistance, repair service and even Zip Code information.

An additional feature is the "Self-Help Guide to Consumer Problems," a separate listing of agencies and organizations which may be of assistance to you.

Here are the area codes for 12 of America's leading cities:

Atlanta, GA 404	Miami, FL 305
Boston, MA 617	New Orleans, LA 504
Chicago, IL 312	New York, NY 212 or 718
Detroit, MI 313	Philadelphia, PA 215
Houston, TX 713	San Francisco, CA 415
Los Angeles, CA 213	Washington, D.C. 202

The first section of the "Yellow Pages" telephone directory contains the following:

1. Information regarding telephone service
2. Business office information
3. Localities served by the particular directory
4. Transit maps
5. Instructions on using, and advertising in, the "Yellow Pages"
6. Telephone tips

This directory lists the commercial establishments in your area according to the type of business organization. In one directory, the following were the first entries: Abattoirs, Abdominal Supports, Abortion and Abortion Alternatives, Abrasives, and Abstracters.

Telephone list, essential. These are the telephone numbers you will use most frequently. It is worthwhile to keep this listing where it is readily available to you.

Police

Fire

Doctor's residence or residences

Answering service

Cleaning service

Hospitals doctor is affiliated with

Pharmacy

Referring doctors

Specialists to whom your doctor refers

Of secondary importance are these numbers:

Accountant

Banks

Building superintendent

Carpenter

Electrician

Equipment repair service

Lawyer

Plumber

Post office

Residences of all office employees

Supply company

Telephone manners. Cultivate a pleasant voice. This can be done by controlling the volume, speaking clearly and not too quickly. Pronounce each word carefully. Above all, *Smile* when you speak. Try to relax and avoid monotony by emphasizing certain words.

Check with your employer. Most dentists prefer to have the secretary use their name in answering the telephone:

"Dr. Jones' office. Good morning. May I help you?"

Be sure that you include some form of greeting in your response. Even if you are harried, do not convey that to the caller, who may feel you are too busy to speak to him or her.

Cordiality is the keynote, and your final words, too, should be cheerful, and include the name of the caller. For example, you might say, "Have a good day," or "It has been nice speaking to you." However, you would never say the latter to someone who is calling because he or she is ill or in pain. In that case be sure to use the "Have a good day" comment.

If you have an office sound system with background music, be sure it is not audible to the caller or interferes with your normal speaking voice.

Toothette (disposable home care device). Your elderly patients may not be capable of brushing their teeth using conventional methods. Toothette is a substitute for both the brush, and, if so desired, for the dentifrice as well. It is a star-shaped piece of polyester foam, at the end of a stick. It is gentle, may be used without water, and is available three ways: with a mint-flavor, nonfoaming dentifrice; premoistened with lime and glycerin for cleaning and soothing teeth and gums, or untreated. It is sold by **Halbrand, Inc.,** Willoughby, OH 44094.

Training new personnel. As people are added to the office staff it is necessary to train them to do things in the manner that they are done in your office. The amount of training necessary will depend on the person's previous experience, but even a person with many years of work in a dental office will need to be shown exactly how they are done in your establishment, and how that person is expected to do them.

Since time and money are expended in training a new staff member, it is important to select wisely from all of the applicants for the job. Once selected and employed, new employees should be given a list of tasks they are expected to perform, and shown, one at a time, how to do them.

Training should never be glossed over. If workers are required to take medical histories, they must be aware of this. If one is required to clean the operatories, it should be made known. If unpleasant tasks are not part of the picture at the very beginning, dissatisfaction comes later on. It is important to train someone slowly and carefully. Never throw too much

196

new material at anyone if he or she is expected to grasp it, and always avoid rushing the process.

It is important that new staff members be welcomed and made to feel at home. This is to your advantage as well, since that new person has been hired to do his or her share of the work in the office.

Make sure no one becomes impatient or bossy with the new person. Above all, treat new workers as the adults they are. When corrections are necessary they should be made quietly and in private, without any shouting. No one takes well to being treated like a child.

It is, of course, bad manners to talk about anyone, but it is especially distressing to new personnel. They should be made to feel they are members of a group which functions as a team.

Never "dump" on the new person all the unpleasant tasks in the office. Where there are a number, share them.

A warm, closely knit unit, with everyone on the staff working together for the common good, benefits everyone.

Tranquil atmosphere. One of the most significant contributions an office manager can make to a busy dental office is to create and maintain a tranquil atmosphere in the reception area. This can be done with care and attention.

No matter how busy or harried the office managers are, they should maintain their "cool." They should never complain to patients about any office procedure or problems. (If an office manager has a complaint, it should be taken to the doctor, so that corrective action may be taken.)

If the office manager's work area is in the reception room, a partial screen may be used to separate it. A three-foot screen, for example, may be used for this purpose. Lamps should be used in the reception area, rather than overhead lights. The use of lamps creates a more homelike atmosphere.

The use of soft music is very valuable in this regard. Also, a soft speaking voice can help a great deal. Even the telephone bell should be kept at the lowest possible volume. It is essential to remember that many patients who come into the office may be upset, and this may manifest itself as anger. Never, ever, allow yourself to get involved in an argument. Remember the patient needs your support and concern. Being friendly and warm can mean a great deal to a person who is in pain. It is important for every member of the office staff to understand the mental anguish patients may be going through.

Today, many office managers are burdened with the task of filling out forms, and it is easy to become annoyed and resentful with patients. However, this should never happen, since supportive behavior is part of the service that must always be available to the patient.

The presence of plants, pictures and photographs—all with an eye to being soothing influences—can help to convey the sought-after feeling of tranquility.

Travel instructions.   Familiarize yourself with travel instructions to your office. These should include how to drive and where to park, and also how to travel by public transportation.

If the office is located in an area which is difficult to reach, you may wish to mimeograph instructions or place them on a business card.

If, when a patient asks instructions, you realize the trip is a long one, tell the patient approximately how much time to allow for it. In this way you can cut down on patient lateness.

Tray systems.   One of the recent developments in dentistry has been the introduction of color-coded trays that are stocked with all instruments needed to perform a given procedure and used as needed. This minimizes time spent setting out materials and instruments, and is far more efficient.

Since instrumentation is an individual choice, it will be up to your employer to specify what should be on the tray.

It is the dental assistant's job, and a vital one, to ensure that there are enough trays set up in advance for whatever procedures are scheduled for the day. You will be able to do this by examining the day sheet, where the procedures to be done are listed.

Until you are confident that you know what will be necessary for each tray, it is a good idea to keep a master list for every procedure your employer does, which you can check before covering the tray. Another alternative is to individually band instruments with a colored plastic ring that corresponds to a given procedure and tray, thereby facilitating an easy set-up.

Typewriter, keeping in good condition. Your typewriter is one of your most-utilized pieces of equipment. To keep it in good working order:

1. Keep it covered when not in use to avoid dust and air pollution.
2. When erasing, move the carriage to the extreme right or left. This prevents the eraser dust from clogging the letters.
3. When oiling, use a very small amount of special oil on the carriage rails, but nowhere else. Use a 3-1 quality oil, but never a heavier one.
4. To clean the type, use a special type cleaner, and a good quality brush.
5. Dust the machine when necessary.
6. Change the typewriter ribbons or cartridge when necessary.
7. Never force a key back into position, or any other part of the typewriter.
8. When the machine requires repair, have the work done by a professional.
9. Try to avoid having others use your typewriter, if at all possible.

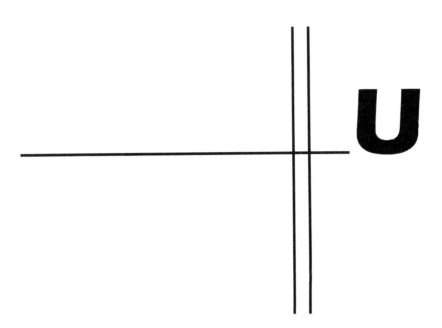

Uniforms. Your uniforms can make you feel great, or mediocre, or smart, or tacky, so it pays to pay attention to its selection and care. (The same, by the way, is true of your makeup and even, to a certain extent, to your shoes.) Because you reflect the way you feel in the way you behave, it is important that you select the type of uniform which expresses your personality—be it chic or casual.

Fortunately, today there are a large variety of uniforms available—with style becoming more and more important. For example, **Diane Von Furstenberg** has designed a collection from which dental assistants may select. You can find full uniforms, as well as "separates" which may be used as summer sportswear because they are so attractive.

Choose your uniforms or outfits as you do your clothes. It is guaranteed you'll spend as much time in them as you do in your "civilian" attire. Find styles which show your figure to its best advantage. Don't settle! The fact that you look well will reflect not only on you, but on the office as well. Take comfort into consideration, too. A too-tight skirt is difficult to sit comfortably in.

Some dentists prefer that their dental assistants dress in white, whereas to others it makes no difference. A bright pink or yellow uniform can actually add to the pleasantness of the office environment.

Heavy jewelry is a no-no, but a choker or small earrings are perfectly suitable.

Your shoes should be comfortable. If you can wear high heels and still run around, there is no reason why you shouldn't. However, if your feet bother you, then your face may reflect the pain, and make it difficult for you to deal with a patient sympathetically.

It goes without saying that everything you wear must be spotless. For that reason, polyester fabrics are a godsend, since they can be washed at night and ready to wear the next morning. Cleanliness is extremely important, and is something that you should always be aware of.

To restore whiteness, use a detergent enhancer such as *Axion*. You'll keep your uniforms white and bright by soaking them in this product. Since *Axion* is not a bleach, it can be used, and will be effective, with colors as well.

Budget Uniform Center, 941 Mill Road, Bensalem, PA., 19025 offers the **Diane Von Furstenberg** collection, plus those of other manufacturers at a 30 percent discount. You may obtain a catalog by writing to them.

Check with **Foley's Uniforms,** 24620 Drake Road, Farmington Hills, MI., 48018. Unusual lab coats, vests and skirts, bib outfits—even a coverall are offered. Colors as well as whites are available, as are designer outfits. Shoes are also offered.

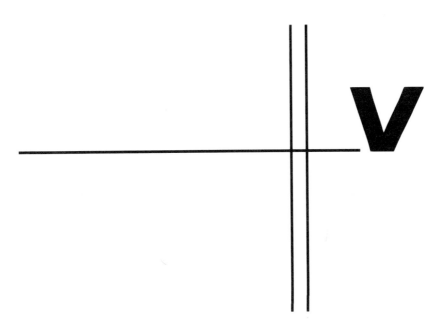

Vital signs. Since dentition is but one facet of a person's health, you may be required to take the vital signs before a patient receives treatment. Vital signs are of value to determine a normal baseline should an emergency ever arise, and also to screen patients for illness they may not be aware of, such as hypertension (high blood pressure), which may be present without any physical symptoms. The vital signs are: temperature, respiration, pulse and blood pressure.

Temperature and respiration are usually considered normal from the onset unless the patient comes in with a head cold or shows visible difficulty in breathing. It is usually safer to reappoint a patient who comes to the office with a cold or a fever, unless the fever is the result of a dental infection, as your entire office and any waiting patients may be incapacitated by the "bug." If the patient insists on being seen, alert the doctor and wear face masks. Patients exhibiting noticeable breathing problems should be referred to a physician; tell your employer if you observe these symptoms.

Pulse rate is taken by palpating (that is, feeling with the first and middle finger) the radial artery, which is located on the thumb side of the inner wrist, or the subclavion artery, which is on the side of the trachea. To locate the subclavion artery, find the long muscle that runs along the side of the neck, and push it back slightly. In both cases, you will feel a series of rhythmic beats. Normal pulse rate is between 60 to 80 beats per minute in adults and between 90 to 100 in children. Elderly patient's average rate is 70 to 80 beats per minute. You can count the number of beats in fifteen seconds and multiply by four to get a pulse rate. Report any abnormality to your doctor and note them on the chart, as well as the date.

Blood pressure is taken using a device called a sphygmomanometer (often shortened to "manometer") and a stethoscope. The Sphygmomanometer is also called a blood pressure cuff, and is placed around the arm above the elbow, with the lower border of the cuff below the crook of the elbow. The cuff must be snug, with no clothing under it. Inflate the cuff after placing the stethoscope under the cuff and checking that you can hear the radial artery. The cuff should be inflated until the sound disappears. Pressure is then slowly released by loosening the valve on the cuff; as the needle or fluid in the gauge begins to fall, a point is reached when you can hear the beats. This is the systolic pressure. As the needle continues to fall, the sounds of the beats get louder, and then gradually decrease in intensity. The weakened beats are heard for a few moments longer, and then they disappear. Complete disappearance of the beats is the point of the diastolic pressure. Normal adult systolic pressure for 20- to 40-year-olds varies from 90 to 140 mm., generally increasing with age. Normal diastolic pressure is 60 to 90mm.

Remember that, for the patient who is anxious, blood pressure may be temporarily elevated. In case you do find a high blood pressure reading, take the pressure in the other arm, or wait 15 minutes and take it again.

Use of an electronic blood pressure machine with a digital reading makes taking the blood pressure almost effortless. You may want to bring this to the attention of your employer.

When a patient has shown an elevated blood pressure, make sure your doctor is aware of this. He or she will probably suggest that patient consult his or her physician.

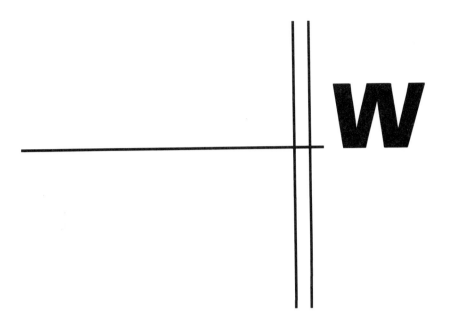

Waiting time, patients. Patients often become irate if they are kept waiting. They become more so if they are being ignored. To avoid this, take into consideration the following:

1. Note the time of arrival for each patient next to his or her name on your list. In that way you can make comments when appropriate, such as, "Mrs. Smith. I realize you've been here for a while. We appreciate your patience."

2. If the doctor has been detained for some reason, inform the patient of this, and let him or her know when the doctor is to be expected.

3. In making appointments, schedule twice as much time for a new patient as you would for a patient making a return visit.

4. When a patient arrives in an emergency situation, he or she must be rushed through. However, it is better to let the other patients know there is an emergency than to have the patients who have been waiting become upset.

5. Do not make light of the delay. Never let a patient think the doctor will see him or her in a few minutes if a longer delay is expected.

Wet weather. During wet weather (primarily winter and spring), it is essential that you have a place to store such things as umbrellas and boots, as well as an absorbent floor mat. By placing the mat right inside the door leading in from the street, you can avoid a wet floor—which is dangerous as well as messy. There should also be a receptacle for both boots and umbrellas for the same purpose. In this way accidents may easily be avoided, and your floor cleaning bills kept down, as well.

An umbrella stand is adequate for umbrellas but doesn't offer a place to store boots. By placing the stand on a large absorbent mat, write a small sign above it saying "Please place your umbrellas and boots here," both items are taken care of.

Hangers for patient's clothing. A place for patients to hang their coats is necessary if your office is in an area where outer garments are necessary.

One of the best types is a metal rod to which the hangers are connected permanently.

Witnessing dental work. As a dental assistant, it is important that you remain in the room while your employer is working on a member of the opposite sex. There have been lawsuits filed against dentists by patients accusing them of sexual advances. This would not have been possible if the assistant was present all of the time the patient was being treated. For example, certain patients may respond to medication by hallucinating, but with a witness in the operatory there is no problem. This rule should be followed especially if the patient is receiving nitrous oxide.

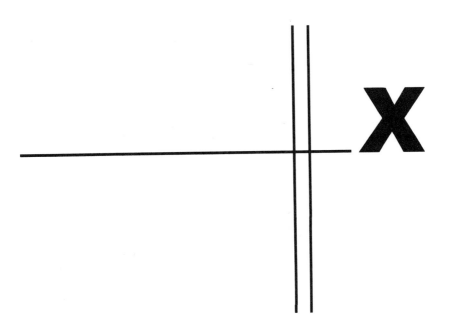

X-rays (radiographs). The safe operation of x-ray equipment is an absolute necessity in the office. Accordingly, the most important factor is the protection of patient and the staff from excessive radiation. The patient is protected by a lead apron or collar shield, which prevents radiation exposure to the thyroid gland. The dental assistant is protected by being outside the room while the x-rays are being taken, or behind a lead barrier. In an era of increasing concern over background radiation, these preventive measures are basic and necessary and demonstrate your care for your patients.

The techniques used in taking radiographs are available from a variety of sources. In general, the two most common types of intraoral x-rays are the "bite wing" and the periapical film. The former enables us to visualize the contact areas of adjacent teeth, and the latter the entire structure of the tooth, it's root and surrounding osseous (bony) structures.

Most offices rely on what is termed a "full series" of x-rays for diagnosing and treatment planning of a new case. The full series must include a bite wing exposure of all posterior teeth (to diagnose proximal caries) and a periapical view of all anterior teeth. The number of exposures needed to obtain a full series can vary depending on film size and operator preference. For recalled patients, the number of films needed will be less, and again, is a matter of the employer's preference.

Periapical films are held in place in the mouth with stabilizers that often provide a target to aim the machine through. Sometimes, the patient's finger may be substituted. Periapical views of anterior teeth are taken with the long sides of the film parallel to the axis of the tooth, and posterior films with the short edges of the film parallel to the roots of the teeth.

Bite wing exposures are taken by using a paper tab to surround the film that should be bitten into by the patient. Again, the short edges of the film packet are parallel to the roots of the teeth. These films may be bent to facilitate easy placement and avoid inpinging on the tongue or the floor or roof of the mouth.

One good rule about patient positioning is the *Up-up-up* rule for lower teeth and the *Down-down-down* rule for upper teeth. That is, for x-rays of the lower teeth, the chair, the patient's chin and the barrel of the x-ray all are in an up position. For the upper dentition, chin, chair and barrel are all pointed downward.

X-ray film packets come in various sizes, including smaller films for children and extra-large sizes for bite wing exposures. These films may have a bite wing tab already present, thereby making use of a paper tab unnecessary.

Developing films is done manually, in a darkroom equipped with metal tubs for developer and fixer, or in an automatic processing machine. Developing films manually is both temperature and time dependent. That is, the length of time the film is immersed in the developer and fixer also depends on the darkroom temperature. The bottles of chemicals used to develop and fix the film have the values used to determine developing time written on them. Keep in mind that film, chemicals and the water used to rinse the developed film are all subject to degradation in time, and must be monitored to insure the best results.

Exposed films may be mounted on special holders for ease of reference. The dental assistant should know how to mount a full series in the format preferred in the office.

X-rays, developing instantly. A new system, *Emmenix Instant Film System*, for developing film in daylight, requires only 20 seconds, and is available at very reasonable cost from **Worldwide Dental, Inc.**, PO Box 14573, St. Petersburg, Florida 33733. It utilizes one solution which both develops and fixes the film. It is possible to code the films as they are being exposed, thereby assuring permanent, positive identification of all negatives. Self-adhesive lead numbers are attached on the outside of the film packets before exposure. A new clipless type of film hanger has also been developed that permits the film to be hung or to stand upright on the side of the container. The film can be placed flat, without touching the surface. Films may be viewed, washed or dried using these hangers.

X-rays, mounting. As mentioned in previous sections, the full-mouth series of radiographs includes periapical views of all teeth, and "bite wings" of all posterior teeth. Periapical exposures of all permanent teeth will need fourteen exposures; bite wing files will take either two or four films, depending on the size film used. Once taken and developed, it will be part of the assistant's duties to mount these films in specially designed mounts.

Films should be mounted to correspond to being viewed from the front; that is, exposures of the right quadrants are mounted to the left of the film holder, and left quadrants on the right.

Full Series of X-Rays, Mounted

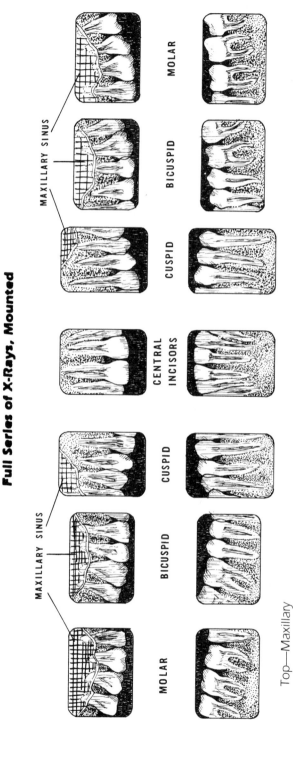

MOLAR

BICUSPID

CUSPID

CENTRAL INCISORS

CUSPID

BICUSPID

MOLAR

MAXILLARY SINUS

MAXILLARY SINUS

MAXILLARY SINUS

MAXILLARY SINUS

Top—Maxillary
Lower—Mandibular
Maxillary sinuses are indicated by crossed lines

210

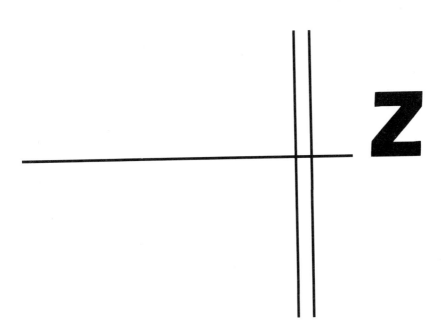

ZIP codes.   In order to have, at your fingertips, a listing of ZIP codes throughout the United States, you should purchase a *National ZIP Code Directory*. It is available, at nominal cost, through your local post office.

Generally, local codes are available in the yellow pages of your telephone directory.

You may also obtain a copy of a local directory, with places within your area, from your post office at a small fee.

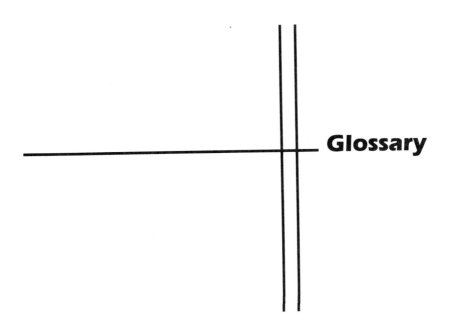

Glossary

abdomen (ăb dō' mĕn). The large body cavity lying below the thorax. It includes the lower portion of the esophagus, the stomach, small and large intestines, liver, gall bladder, pancreas, spleen and urinary bladder.

abduct (ăb dŭkt'). To move away from the midline of the body.

ablation (ăb lā' shŭn). Removal; excision—amputation.

abrasion (ăb rā' zhŭn). Scraped area of skin or mucous membrane.

abrasive (ă brā' siv). Polishing and grinding agent used to reduce cast metal, composite, porcelain or amalgam.

abscess (ăb' sĕs). Infection which may be found at root tip or on side (lateral) of tooth. It is a localized collection of pus in

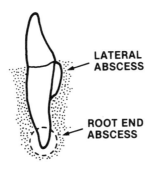

LATERAL
ABSCESS

ROOT END
ABSCESS

213

body tissues, usually caused by bacteria. Dental abscesses are caused by cariously infected teeth, or by periodontal (gum) disease. Usually if the abscess channels through the surrounding bone and soft tissue there is little pain.

abutment (á bŭt' mĕnt). In prosthetics, a tooth used to support replacement teeth in a denture or a bridge.

acapnia (a kăp' ni a). Absence of carbon dioxide in the blood.

acephalous (a sĕf' a lŭs). Minus a head.

acetaminophen (a set a min' o fen). A pain killer containing no salicylates (e.g. aspirin).

acetone (ăs' e tōn). Inflammable solvent with characteristic odor.

acetylcholine (ăs et il kō' len). A chemical released from nerve endings that activates muscle, gland and other nerve cells.

achalasia (ăk a lā' zhi a). Failure to relax.

acid etch (ăs' id ĕch). A technique of roughening enamel to produce more retention for a filling. A 50 percent phosphoric acid solution is applied topically, then washed off.

acidosis (aš id ō' sis). Depletion of carbonates in the blood causing an acid base imbalance.

acne (ăk' nē). A common condition in adolescents in which blackheads are associated with pustular eruptions of the skin; an inflamatory disease of the sebaceous glands.

acrocephalia (ăk rō se fā' li a). A congenital malformation in which the top of the head is pointed.

acrodynia (ăk rō din' i a). In children a painful reddening of the extremities (Synonym: Swift's Disease).

acromegaly (ak' rō mĕg' a li). A pituitary disturbance causing enlarged hands, feet and face.

acrylic (a kril' ik). Plastic-like material used as a denture base, temporary filling or crown, or as a facing on a cast crown.

actinomyces (ăk ti nō mī̄ sēz). Parasitic fungus characterized by radiating filaments.

acuity (a kū' i ti). Sharpness; keenness (e.g. visual acuity).

acupuncture (ak' ū pŭngk tur). The insertion of special needles into parts of the body for the treatment of disease, pain relief or to produce anesthesia.

acute caries (a kūt' kar' i ez). Condition associated with presence of multiple cavities; often found in children.

ADA. Abbreviation for **American Dental Association**.

adaptic (ā dap' tik). Nongeneric name for a composite filling material.

addict (ăd' ikt). A person who cannot resist indulgence in some habit. Usually, withdrawal causes severe trauma.

Addison's disease (Ad' di sonz di zēz'). Deficiency in secretions of the adreno-cortex causing lowered blood pressure and blood volume; brownish pigmentation of skin and anemia.

adduction (ăd dŭk' shŭn). The act of drawing towards the midline of the body.

adenitis (ad' en ī' tis). Inflammation of a lymph node or gland.

adenoid (ăd' ě noid). An enlarged mass of lymphoid tissue in the upper pharynx.

adenoma (ăd e nō' ma). A benign tumor of glandlike structure.

adenopathy (ad en op' a thi). A disease of a gland, usually lymphatic.

adhesion (ăd hē' zhŭn). Abnormal union of adjacent tissues common after inflammation.

adipose (ăd' i pōz). Fat.

adnexa (ăd něk' sa). Structures in close proximity to a part.

adrenalin (ăd rěn' al in). Hormone produced by the medulla of the adrenal gland.

adrenergic (ăd ren er' jik). Referring to sympathetic nerves that liberate adrenalin from their ends. Opposite of cholinergic.

adventitia (ăd věn tish' i a). The outside covering of an artery or vein.

aerobe (ā' er ōb). A microorganism which needs air, particulary oxygen, for life.

aerophagia (ă' ĕr ō fā' jia). Excessive swallowing of air.

afebrile (ā fĕb' rĭl). Without fever.

agenesis (a jĕn' e sis). Incomplete development, such as the absence of a limb.

agglutination (ă glooō' ti nā shun). The clumping of bacteria or blood cells due to the action of antibodies called agglutinins.

aglossia (a glŏs' i a). Absence of a tongue.

agranulocyte (a grăn' ū lo sit). A white blood cell without granules.

albamycin (al ba mī' sin).An antibiotic; its generic name is novobiccin.

aldosterone (ăl dŏs' ter ōn). An adreno-cortical hormone that regulates potassium and sodium metabolism.

alginate (ăl ji' nāt). Material made from marine kelp; used to take impressions of the mouth and teeth.

alimentary (al' i mĕn' ta ri). Pertaining to nutrition.

alkali (ăl ka lĭ). Any of the various chemical basis, the hydroxides, which neutralize acids to form a salt and water.

alkaloid (ăl' ka loid). A large group of organic bases found in plants, that possess important physiological powers. They include nicotine, morphine, caffeine and strychnine.

allergen (ăl' er jĕn). Any substance capable of producing an allergic reaction.

allergy (ăl' er ji). A hypersensitivity (such as hay fever or asthma) to certain things such as pollen; characterized by difficulty in respiration and/or skin rashes.

allograft (ăl' lo graft). The transplantation of a part from one person to another. It may be skin or an organ.

alloy (ă loi'). Metallic substance consisting of two or more metals melted together. The commonest alloy used in dentistry—amalgam—is alloyed via the process known as trituration.

alopecia (al' o pē' shia). Baldness.

alphosyl (al' fo sl). A colorless derivative of coal tar used to treat psoriasis and other skin diseases.

216

alveolus (ăl vē' o lus). **1.** An air cell of the lung. **2.** A socket of a tooth.

amalgam (a mal' gam). Alloy of mercury, silver, copper and tin used to fill teeth.

ambulatory (am' bū la tō ri). Able to walk.

ameloblastoma (a mē' lō' blăs tō mă). Tumor of the tooth germ (adamantinoma).

ametropia (ăm' e trō' pi ă). Poor sight due to the faulty refraction of light waves by the eye.

amino acids (ă mī' no ăs' idz). Organic acids that are the end product of protein metabolism.

ammonium chloride (am mō' ni ŭm chlo' rīd). **1.** A chemical used to treat urinary infections. **2.** Also used as a mild expectorant.

amnesia (ăm nē zhi a). Loss of memory, either partial or complete.

amphetamine (ăm fet' a mēn). A powerful stimulant of the central nervous system used to treat depression, and as an appetite depressant.

ampicillin (ăm pi sil' lin). A broad-spectrum antibiotic given orally or by injection.

ampule (ăm pūl). A small, sealed glass vial containing a single drug dose. Unlike a carpule, which is inserted into a syringe and then injected, the contents of the ampule must be retracted into the syringe and then discarded.

anaerobe (ăn aer' ōb). A bacteria that does not require an environment containing oxygen.

analgesia (ăn ăl jē'zi a). Loss of pain.

analgesic (an al jē' sik). A drug causing loss of pain.

anaphylaxis (ăn' a fi lak' sis). The most severe form of allergic response to a foreign substance. It may cause suffocation due to swelling of the respiratory passages. If this occurs, a tracheotomy must be performed to allow respiration.

anaplasia (ăn a plā' zhi a). A cell or cells that have lost anatomical characteristics normal to appearance; usually associated with cancer.

anastomosis (an as to mō' sis). Connection between parts of any two organs or branches of a system, such as blood vessels.

Anatomy of tooth (a nat' a mē).

Crown—exposed part of tooth

Root—portion of tooth imbedded in bone

Apex—tip of root

Enamel—outer covering of tooth–hardest substance in the body.

Dentin—portion of tooth lying beneath enamel–softer and more sensitive

Pulp—usually called "nerve"–in the center of tooth. Actually made up of nerves, blood vessels and other tissue.

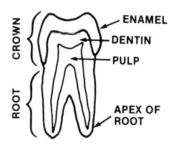

anemia (ă nē' mi a). An illness caused by a deficiency in numbers of red blood cells and/or their hemoglobin content.

anesthesia (an es thē' zhi a). Local or general insensibility to pain, induced by specific drugs or by nerve damage.

aneurysm (ăn' u riz m). A permanent weakening and swelling of a blood vessel due to a local fault in its wall through birth, disease or injury.

angiectasis (an ji ek' ta sis). An abnormal enlargement of blood vessels.

angiitis (an gi ī' tis). An inflammation of a blood or lymph vessel.

angina (an jī' na). A temporary painful attack of cardiac discomfort that may radiate to the arms; usually induced by exercise.

angioma (an ji ō' ma). A benign tumor consisting of blood vessels.

angioneurotic edema (an ji ō nū rŏt' ik ē dē' ma). Severe swelling involving skin of hands, face, or genitals and/or mucous membranes of mouth or throat. May be due to allergy; often no cause can be found.

anhydrous (ăn hī' drus). Lacking water; dry.

ankylosis (ang ki lō' sis). The union of two or more bones or joints into one.

ankyloglossia (ang' ki lŏ glos' si a). Abnormal attachment of tongue to floor of mouth (tongue-tie).

anneal (a nēl'). To place a metal under high heat to burn off impurities. This is most commonly performed when placing direct gold fillings, either on a heated tray or, with cohesive gold, directly over a flame while holding the gold with an explorer.

anodontia (ăn o don' shi a). Absence of teeth.

anodyne (an' ō' dīn). Pain-relieving remedy.

anomaly (a nŏm' a li). A clincal observation of anything unusual or abnormal, such as a supernumerary (extra) tooth.

anorectic (an o rek' tik). An appetite depressent.

anorexia (ăn o reks' i a). Loss of appetite for food.

anosomia (ăn ŏz' mi a). Missing the sense of smell.

anoxia (ăn ok' si a). Lack of oxygen in tissues.

antemortem (ăn tī mor' tĕm). Just before death.

anterior (ăn tēr' i er). Descriptive term meaning "in front." The anterior teeth are the two incisors and cuspids in the upper and lower jaws.

anteversion (an' tē ver' zhun). Forward tilt of an organ or part.

antibiotic (an' ti bī ot' ik). An agent produced by fungi or bacteria that destroys other bacteria.

antibody (an' ti bod ē). A protein found in the blood serum which is produced in response to stimuli in the blood.

antiemetic (an' ti e met' ik). An agent that prevents vomiting.

antifebrile (an ti fĕb' ril). An agent which combats fever.

antihistamine (an' ti hist' a mēn). A drug which inhibits the effects of released histamine, used in the treatment of hay fever and other allergies.

antiphlogistic (an' ti flō jis' tik). An inflammation-relieving agent.

antipruritic (an' ti proo rit' ik). A substance that prevents or relieves itching.

antipyretic (an ti pī rĕt' ik). A substance that reduces fever.

antiscorbutic (an' ti skōr bu' tik). Any substance that prevents scurvy; specifically vitamin C.

antiseptic (an ti sep' tik). Any substance that destroys or interferes with the growth or microorganisms.

antisialagogue (an ti sī' al ă gŏg). Any substance that slows down salivation.

antispasmodic (an ti spaz mod' ik). Any substance that may be used to relieve muscle spasm.

antithrombin (an ti throm' bin). Any substance occurring naturally in the blood that inhibits clotting.

antitoxin (an ti tok' sin). An agent manufactured in the body in response to bacterial invasion or by injection of a dose of treated toxin. The agent neutralizes a specific toxin.

antitussive (an ti tus' iv). A cough suppressant; cough suppressing measures.

antrostomy (an tros' tomi). An artifical opening created between the nasal cavity and the maxillary sinus, to produce drainage.

anus (ā' nus). Distal end of the alimentary canal.

aorta (ā or' ta). The major artery coming out of the left ventricle of the heart.

APC. Aspirin, phenacetin and caffeine together in tablet form. Used as a pain killer.

apex (ā' peks). The top of any cone-shaped structure. In dentistry, the tip of the root of a tooth.

apexification (a' peks if i kā shun). Technique used to promote the termination of growth of the tooth's root to enable a root canal to be finished.

aphagia (a fā' ji a). The inability to swallow.

aphasia (a fā' zhi a). A speech disorder caused by a brain lesion.

aphthae (af' thē). Small gray-colored areas surrounded by a reddish ring that occur in the mouth.

apicoectomy (ap' i kō ĕk tō mi). Surgical procedure to remove root-end abcess. The dentist will go through bone and eliminate infection physically. Usually includes removing infected root tip and packing wound with antibiotics.

aplasia (ā plā' zhia). Defective growth or development of an organ or tissue.

apnea (ăp nē' a). A temporary stopping of breathing.

apophysis (ap of' is is). A protuberance or outgrowth, usually of bone.

aqueous (ā' kwē ŭs). Watery; containing water.

arachnoid (a rak' noid). Resembling a spider's web; the membrane covering the brain and spinal cord.

arginine (ar ji nen). One of the essential amino acids.

Aristocort (a ris' tō kort). An antiinflammatory steroid; generic name is triamcinolone.

arrhythmia (ā rith' mi a). A deviation from the normal rhythm, usually of the heart.

arteriogram (ar te' ri ō gram). An X-ray film that shows the arteries after the injection of opaque dye.

arteriosclerosis (ar te' ri ō skle rō sis). A degenerative hardening of arteries usually occuring with advanced age.

arteritis (ar ti rī' tis). Inflammation of an artery.

arthralgia (arth ral' ji a). Joint pain usually with no inflammation.

arthrectomy (ar threk' tō mi). Surgical removal of a joint.

arthritis (ar thrī' tis). Inflammation of a joint.

arthrogram (arth rō' gram). An X-ray film that demonstrates the state of health of the joint.

articulation (ar tik ū lā' shun). The junction of two or more bones, as in a joint.

articulator (ar tik' ū lā' tor). Mechanical device used to fabricate dentures or crowns by allowing stone models to be set in duplication of a patient's natural jaw position.

asbestos (ăs bĕs' tŏs). A fibrous mineral substance used in making protective heat-resistant products.

ascorbic acid (a skor' bik as' id). Vitamin C.

asepsis (ā sep' sis). An enviroment free of disease-causing microorganisms.

asphyxia (as fik' si a). Cessation of breathing; suffocation.

aspiration (as pi rā' shun). 1. To withdraw fluids from a body cavity by siphonage or suction. 2. Breathing in. 3. A goal. 4. Technique used in obtaining local anesthesia via injection.

asthenia (as thē' ni a). Weakness; a state of being debilitated.

asthma (az' ma). Obstruction of the air passages caused by narrowing of the bronchi. It is a reversible condition.

astigmatism (a stig' ma tizm). Defective vision caused by unequal refractive surfaces of the cornea.

astringent (as trin' jent). Any substance that causes tissue to shrink or contract.

ataractic (at a rak' tik) Drugs that relieve anxiety without causing drowsiness.

ataxia (ā tak' si a). Irregular movement due to poor muscle control.

atheroma (ath e rō ma). 1.Deposits of fat in the inner linings of the arterial walls. 2. A type of sebaceous cyst.

atonic (a ton' ik). Weak; without muscular tension.

atopy (at' ōp i). Familial allergy.

atresia (a tre' zhi a). Abnormal closure of an opening.

atrial fibrillation (a' tri al fib ril ā' shun). Wild cardiac irregularity.

atrial flutter (ā' tri ăl flut' er). Regular, fast cardiac rhythm.

atrial septal defect (ā' tri al sep' tal dē' fekt). A congenital heart defect caused by nonclosure of the foramen ovale.

atromid (at' rō mid). A drug that lowers blood cholesterol.

atrophy (at' ro fī). Wasting; decrease in size and function.

atropine (at' ro pēn). Chief alkaloid of belladonna, which is a central nervous system depressant and which decreased secretions of the bronchial and salivary systems.

audiology (aw di ol' o ji). Science of the study of hearing.

auditory (aw' di tō ri). Relating to the sense of hearing.

aura (aw' ra). A warning or premonition of an impending attack such as epilepsy.

autism (aw' tizm). A childhood syndrome involving extreme withdrawal from reality.

autoclave (aw' tō klāv). An apparatus for sterilization using high-pressure steam.

autogenous (aw toj' e nus). Self-produced; usually refers to skin or bone graft, using the patient's own tissues.

autolysis (aw tol' īs is). Self-digestion; occures when digestive juices escape into surrounding tissues.

autometism (aw tom' at izm). Performing of involuntary acts (e.g. epilepsy, somnambulism).

autonomic (aw tō nom' ik). Self-governing; specifically the autonomic nervous system, which is made up of nerve cells and fibers that act involuntarily.

autopsy (aw' top si). Examination of a body after death.

avitaminosis (a vīta min ōs' is). A disease caused by vitamin deficiency.

avulsion (a vul' shun). Forcible tearing or wrenching away.

axial (ak si al). Descriptive term for axis of a part. In dentistry, it refers to the longest plane of the tooth in an "up-down" configuration.

axon (ak' son). The part of the nerve fiber that carries impulses away from the cell.

bacillus (ba sil' us). A type of bacteria consisting of aerobic rod-shaped cells, gram positive, producing endospores.

bacitracin (ba sĕ trā sin). An antibiotic used externally.

bacteremia (băk te rē' mi a). The presence of bacteria in the blood.

bacteria (băk tēr' i a). Small cells, which may be spherical, straight rods, curved rods or spirals. They may cause disease, fermentation or putrefaction. They are plant cells, having a cell wall, as well as a cell membrane and nucleus. Other structures such as capsules or flagella may be present.

bactericide (bak tēr' i sīd). Any bacterial-destroying agent.

bacteriolysis (bak tēr i ō' līs is). The disintegration of bacteria.

bacteriophage (bak ter' i ō făj). A virus that lives on bacteria, thereby destroying them.

barbiturates (bar bit' ū rātz). A group of drugs used as sedatives derived from barbituric acid.

basal ganglia (bā' sal gang' li a). A collection of gray nerve cells at the base of the cerebrum which modify and coordinate voluntry muscle movement.

basal metabolism (bā' sal met a' bōl izm). The amount of energy required to maintain life in a resting state.

basal narcosis (bās' sal nar kō' sis). The administration, before anesthesia, of drugs that reduce anxiety and induce sleep.

base (bās). 1.That part of a filling that is placed under the silver to insulate or medicate the tooth. 2. The part of a denture that rests on soft tissue.

basophil (bā' so fil). A substance that takes up dyes; usually used to refer to certain white blood cells.

Bass Method (Băs mĕth' ŭd). Tooth brushing technique in which bristles are placed at 45° angle between tooth and gum and overlapping horizontal strokes are employed.

battered baby syndrome (băt' ĕrd bā' bi sin' drōm). An infant that exhibits physical injuries, usually to the head, extremities, chest or long bones, and that can't be explained by natural disease or accidents.

BCG (Bacillus—Calmette—Guerin). A vaccine used to immunize against tuberculosis.

224

Bead Sterilizer (Bēd Ster' i līz' er). Used in endodontic therapy to render instruments free from germs. Uses hot glass beads.

belladonna (běl a don' a). A strong antispasmodic made from dried leaves of the nightshade (a plant).

Bell's Palsy (Belz Pawl' zi). Paralysis of half the face due to swelling of the seventh cranial nerve.

Benadryl (běn a dril). Diphenhydroamine; an antihistaminic drug.

benzedrine (ben zē drin). An amphetamine.

benzocaine (ben' zō kān). A surface anesthetic.

beri-beri (běr' ē běr' ē). A deficiency disease caused by lack of Vitamin B_1 (thiamin).

bevel (běv el). A slope. Preparations for crowns or inlays are beveled to provide a finishing line closest to the contour of the original tooth, thus minimizing gingival irritation.

bicarbonate (bī kar' bŏn āt). A carbonic-acid salt; when present in the blood indicates the alkaline reserve.

biconcave (bī kon' kāv). Hollow on both surfaces.

biconvex (bī kon' veks). Bulging on both surfaces.

bifid (bī fid). Forked.

bifurcation (bī fur kā' shun). Divided into two branches. In dentistry refers especially to area where roots of posterior teeth divide.

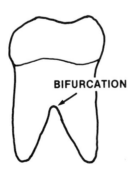

BIFURCATION

bilateral (bī lat' er al). Pertaining to both sides.

bile (bīl). A heavy, greenish-colored alkaline fluid secreted by the liver and stored in the gall bladder.

biopsy (bī' op si). The removal of a piece of living tissue for histologic examination. Biopsies are commonly done on any abnormal growth encountered in the mouth and on deep-seated infections at the apex of teeth. The three commonest techniques are excision, punch biopsy or exfoliative cytology.

biotin (bī' ot in). One of the B complex vitamins.

biparous (bip' ar us). Bring forth offspring in pairs.

bisexual (bī sek' shoo ăl). 1. Having both male and female characteristics. 2. Sexually responsive to both sexes.

biteplate (bīt' plāt). An acrylic appliance used to correct occlusal discrepancies by covering the biting surfaces of the teeth to prevent overclosure. They are often made to be worn at night.

bite wing (bīt' wing). The paper holder used with X-ray film to photograph the interproximal area of the teeth. The patient bites the paper tab to insure proper placement of the film. This technique is used for the posterior teeth.

Black, G.V. (1836-1915). "Father" of modern dentistry. His techniques and instruments for cavity preparation are still taught and used.

Black hairy tongue (Blăk har' ē tung). Condition in which filiform papillae of tongue are stained.

bleb (blĕb). A large blister or vesicle filled with fluid.

blepharitis (blef a rī' tis). Inflammation of the eyelid.

blood (blud). The thick red fluid that travels through the heart, filling the blood vessels. It consists of a colorless fluid called *plasma,* within which blood cells, or *corpuscles,* plus minute round bodies called *platelets,* are suspended.
There are red corpuscles, call *erythrocytes,* and white corpuscles, called *leukocytes.* In the normal state there are approximately 4.5 million to 5 million red blood cells (abbreviated r.b.c.) per cubic millimeter of blood, and from 5 thousand to 10 thousand white blood cells per cubic millimeter.

blood count (blud kount). The calculation of the number of red or white blood cells per cubic millimeter of blood using an instrument called a hemocytometer.

blood cross matching (blud kros maching). The testing of the compatability of samples of blood from two different people, which must be done before a transfusion.

blood culture (blud kul' tur). A test to determine the presence of any microorganisms in the sample of blood.

blood group (blud groop). There are two basic systems.
In the ABO system there are four groups; A, B, AB and O. The groups are determined by the presence of different antigens. These groups are important in determining whether or not it is possible to transfuse blood from one person to another.
In the *Rhesus,* or rh blood-grouping system there are other antigens that are important in the determination of fetal blood compatability with that of the mother. Human blood is either rh positive or rh negative.

blood pressure. The pressure exerted by the flow of blood on blood vessel walls. It is measured in millimeters of mercury, using a sphygmomanometer. When the heart muscle is at its maximum contraction it is recorded first; this is the systolic pressure. When the left ventricle of the heart is relaxed, this is the diastolic pressure.

Blood sedimentation rate (BSR) (blud sed i měn tā' shun rāt). A test performed on a blood sample to determine the presence of inflammation in the body.

blood sugar (blud shoog' er). The amount of glucose present in the circulating blood.

B.M.R. Basal metabolic rate.

boil (boil). An acute inflammation of a hair follicle caused by the bacterium Staphylococcus aureus.

bolus (bō' lus). A pulpy soft lump of masticated food.

bonding (bond ēng). Cosmetic process used to apply facings or composites to the teeth.

bone (bōn). The hard tissue that forms the skeleton.

bone graft (bōn graft). The transplanting of a piece of bone from one person to another or from one part of the body to another.

bradycardia (brad' i kar' di a). A slow pulse rate caused by a slow heart-contraction rate.

brain (brān). The part of the central nervous system that is located in the cranial cavity, or skull. It is divided into the cerebrum, cerebellum, pons variolii, midbrain and medulla oblongata.

Brevitol (brev' i tol). A barbiturate that has no sulfur.

bridge (brij). In dentistry, a bridge is a means of replacing a lost tooth by using adjacent teeth for support.

Bright's disease (brīts di zēz'). Kidney inflammation or nephritis.

bromides (brō' midz). A group of drugs containing bromine salts which act as mild central nervous system depressants.

bromism (brō' mizm). Chronic poisoning caused by excessive use of bromides.

bronchi (bron' kī). The two (2) tubes into which the lower end of the trachea divides, and which then divide further in the lung.

bronchiectasis (brŏng ki ek' ta sis). Dilation of the bronchi following lung infection.

bronchiole (brong' ki ōl). One of the tiny subdivisions of the bronchi at its termination in the air sacs of the lung.

bronchitis (bron kī' tis). An inflammation of the bronchi characterized by wheezing, breathlessness and a productive cough.

bronchogenic (brong kō jen' ik). Arising from, or caused by, the bronchi.

bronchoscope (brong' kō skōp). An instrument used to examine the inside of the bronchi.

brux. To clench.

bruxism (bruks' izm). Condition where patient clenches and grinds teeth, often while sleeping. Therapy can involve an acrylic bite plate.

bubo (bū bō). Swollen lymph glands, usually in the groin.

buccal (buk' al). Descriptive term referring to cheek and mouth. The buccal surface of teeth lies closest to the cheek and lips.

Buerger's disease (ber' gers di zez'). A disease in which the peripheral blood vessels are obliterated.

bulbar (bul' bar). Referring to the medulla oblongata.

bulla (bool' a). A large watery blister.

B.U.N. The amount of urea present in circulating blood (Blood Urea Nitrogen). This rises in kidney disease.

bur (bŭr). The bit that is used in a dental handpiece. Burs are available in a variety of shapes and sized for both the slow- and high-speed drills.

burnish (bur' nish). To rub the surface of a silver filling to bring oxides to the surface of the silver, thereby strengthening the restoration. This is performed directly after condensing the amalgam in the cavity.

burnisher (bur' nish er). Instrument used to burnish a filling.

Burrows Solution (bur' oz so lū shŭn). An antiseptic solution of aluminum acetate.

bursa (bur' sa). A fibrous sac containing fluid.

bursitis (bur sī' tis). An inflamed bursa.

butabarbital (būt a barb' itol). Butisol. A moderately rapid and strong hypnotic.

butacaine (bū' ta kān). A synthetic surface anesthetic used in ophthalmology.

cachexia (ka kek' si a). A physical state of ill health including malnutrition, emaciation and dull-looking eyes.

cadaver (ka dav' er). A dead body.

caffeine (kaf' ē in). A stimulant found in tea and coffee.

calcareous (kal ka' ri us). Containing calcium or lime.

calcium (kal' sī um). A metallic element found in food. It is essential for health of the bones, teeth, blood and enzyme systems.

calcium hydroxide (kal' sē um hī drok sīd). Commonly used base for a filling that causes secondary dentin growth.

calculus (kal' kū lus). A hard, abnormal mineral substance found in body cavities and on the teeth. Calculus is formed when the bacteria in plaque are not removed by brushing or flossing. (See Illustration page 230.)

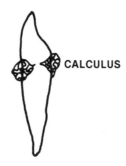

CALCULUS

Caldwell-Luc operation (cald wel luk). A technique for opening and draining the maxillary sinus in the area of the upper bicuspid teeth.

caliper (kal' ip er). 1. A two-pronged instrument for measurement of diameter. 2. A double-pronged instrument used in the fixation of long bones.

callus (kal' us). The calcified tissue that forms at the end of fractured bones and helps in their repair.

calorie (kal' o rē). The amount of heat necessary to raise the temperature of one gram of water one degree centigrade.

calvarium (kal va' ri um). The top or vault of the skull.

camphor (kam' for). A solid, white, pungent-smelling substance used in cough mixtures and, externally, in oils as an analgesic.

cancellous (kan' sell us). A spongy latticework structure.

cancer (kan' ser). A general term used to identify malignant growths in all parts of the body.

cancrumoris (kang krum o'ris). A destructive inflammation of the mucosa of the mouth, seen in debilitated children.

candida (kan' di da). A fungus found in many parts of the body.

canines (kā' nīnz). Teeth that, used with incisors, bite into food. They (named from the word "canine" or "dog" because they resemble the dog's fangs) are also used to tear food. They have a sharp edge and one root.

canker (kang' ker). White lesions found on the oral mucosa. These lesions, which are very common, are also known as "cold sores."

cannula (kan' ū la). A hollow tube used to withdraw from or introduce fluid into the body.

cantharides (kan thar' i dēz). A blistering agent made from dried Spanish beetles.

canthus (kan' thus). The angles formed by the junction of the eyelids with the face. Used in cephalometrics as an easily identified landmark.

capillary (kap' i lar i). A thin-walled tiny blood vessel which lies between the ends of the arteries and the beginnings of the veins. It aids in the rapid exchange of substances from the blood stream and the surrounding tissue.

capsule (kap' sūl). A thin outer covering of organs like the liver, spleen and kidney.

Carabelli's cusp (Kar a beliz kusp). Condition where a molar tooth has prominent extra cusp.

carbocaine (kar' bō kan). Mepivacaine. A local anesthetic that is manufactured without epinephrine.

carbohydrate (kar bō hī' drāt). An organic compound containing carbon, oxygen, and hydrogen; found in sugars and starches, these are important source of energy in man.

carbolic acid (kar bŏl' ik as' id). Phenol.

carboxyhemoglobin (kar boks' i hēm ō glō' bin). A chemical formed by the union of hemoglobin from the red cells, and carbon monoxide.

carbuncle (kar' bung kl). A painful inflammation of the subcutaneous tissue similar to, but more serious than a boil, involving hair follicles that result in suppuration and sloughing.

carcinogen (kar si' nō gen). A cancer-producing agent or substance.

carcinoma (kar si nō' ma). A malignant and invasive tumor of epidermoid tissues; cancer.

cardiac (kar' di ak). Pertaining to the heart or the cardia.

cardiogram (kar' di ō gram).A recording of the form and force of the heartbeat.

cardiovascular (kar dī ō vas' kul ar). Relating to the heart and blood vessels.

carditis (kar dī tis). Inflammation of the membranes of the heart, either pericardium, endocardium or myocardium.

caries (kăr' ēz). Process of decalcification of teeth; lay term is "decay." Caries is a multifactorial disease caused by the interaction of the host's resistance, the bacteria that causes decay, and the carbohydrates in the diet that the bacteria live on.

carotid (kar' ot' id). A major artery found on each side of the neck.

cartilage (kar' ti laj). Tough connective tissue.

cascara (kas kar' a). An extract of bark used as a purgative.

caseation (ka zi ā' shun). The formation of a cheesy, soft mass.

cast (kast). Laboratory process used to make metal prostheses.

catabolism (ka tab' ō lizm). The breakdown of food substances taken into the body into simple chemicals plus the release of energy.

catalyst (kat' a list). An agent that speeds up a chemical reaction without undergoing any change itself.

catarrh (ka tar'). An inflammation of a mucous membrane accompanied by a heavy flow of mucus.

catheter (kath' e ter). A hollow tube of various lengths and diameters used to introduce or withdraw fluids from the body cavities.

caudal block (kaw' dal blok). Injection of local anesthetic in the caudal area.

caustic (kaws' tik). An agent that is destructive to organic tissues.

cautery (kaw' ter i). A caustic agent, usually a heated metal point or wire.

cauterize (kaw' ter īz). The process of using a heated metal point or wire to either remove tissue or stop hemorrhage.

The machine employed in dentistry to accomplish this is often called an *electrosurge*.

cavernous (kav' er nus). A hollow space or channel.

cavity (kav' i tē). Hollow place synonymous with tooth
decalcification.

cavity classification (kav i tē klas i fi kā shun). Accepted means
of charting location on the tooth structure where the cavity
appears.

Class I—cavity is on biting surface of a posterior tooth.

Class II—cavity is on interproximal surface; that is, where
two teeth meet.

Class III—Cavity is on the proximal surface of an anterior
tooth not involving the incisal (corner) angle of the
tooth.

Class IV—cavity is on proximal of an anterior and involves
the incisal angle.

Class V—cavity is on gingival third of tooth.

cellulitis (sel' u lī' tis). Inflammation of tissue.

cement (se ment'). Material commonly used as a base under
deep fillings. It protects the pulp from irritation caused by
the restoration and "hot and cold."

cementoma (se men' tō ma). Growth (abnormal) of cementum
which in effect ankyloses (fuses) tooth to socket.

cementum (se men' tum). Natural substance that covers the
dentin in the root of the tooth, and anchors the tooth to the
socket below the gumline.

cephalometrics (sef' a lō met' riks). In orthodonture, study of
facial growth using multiple X-rays and tracings to monitor
development of teeth.

ceramic (se ram' ik). In dentistry, refers to porcelain part of a
crown, or inlay.

cervical (sur' vi kal). Relating to the neck.

chancre (shang' ker). An ulcer, one type of which is found is
primary syphilis.

chancroid (shang' kroid). A veneral disease usually found in the tropics, characterized by painful ulcers on the penis and vulva.

chart (chart). 1. Record on which clinical findings and treatments are recorded. 2. Process of examining and transfering data to the record.

cheilitis (kī lī' tis). Irritation and cracking of the corners of the mouth.

cheilosis (kī lō' sis). Irritation and cracking of the corners of the mouth.

chemotherapy (kēm ō ther' ap i). Treatment of disease with specific chemical agents that do not permanently injure healthy tissue.

chloral hydrate (klor' al hī' drāt). Quick-acting sedative and hypnotic.

Chloramphenicol (klor am fen' ik ol). An orally administered broad-spectrum antibiotic that may cause aplastic anemia.

chloroform (klor' ō form). A heavy liquid once widely used as an anesthetic.

chlorpromazine (klor prō' ma zēn). A widely used drug with antispasmodic, sedative and hypotensive properties. Its most frequent use is in psychiatric and geriatric patients.

cholera (kol' e ra). A serious epidemic disease mostly found in the Eastern nations, caused by Vibriocholera bacteria.

cholesterol (kōl es ter al). A fatty crystalline substance, manufactured in the body, and found in the blood, nerve tissues and liver. It crystallizes along the walls of arteries. It also occurs in animal and dairy foods.

choline (kō' lēn). A chemical found in animal tissues and involved in the growth and transportation of fats, within the body.

cholinergic (kōl in er' jik). Referring to parasynthetic nerves which liberate acetylcholine.

chondritis (kon drī' tis). Inflammation of cartilage.

chondroma (kon drō' ma). A benign cartilage tumor.

chondrosarcoma (kon drō sar kō' ma). A malignant tumor of cartilage.

chorditis (kor dī' tis). Inflammation of either the vocal or spermatic cords.

chorea (kō rē a). A neural disease characterized by jerky, spasmodic, uncontrollable movements.

chromatography (krō ma tog' ra fi). The separation of mixtures into their constituents on a chromatograph column.

chomosome (krō' mō sōm). Any of several threadlike bodies, found in a cell nucleus, that carry the hereditary factors or genes.

chyme (kīm). The partially digested mass of food that passes from the stomach to the small intestine.

cicatrix (sik' a triks). A connective tissue scar.

cilia (sil' i a). Tiny, hairlike processes which extend from the surface of cells.

cimex (sī meks). A genus of insects including the common bedbug.

circadian rhythm (ser' kā dī an rith'm). Rhythmic cycles recurring at 24-hour intervals.

cirrhosis (si rō sis). Degenerative hardening of a body organ, usually the liver.

cirsoid (sur' soid). Enlargement of a vein.

cleft palate (kleft pal' it). Congential incomplete fusion of the two halves of the palatal bone.

cleidocranial dysostosis (kli dō krā' nē al dīsōs to' sis). Congential disease associated with delayed eruption of permanent teeth.

cleocin (klē ō sin). An active antibiotic. Clindamycin.

clofibrate (klō fib' rāt). A drug used to lower blood cholesterol.

clonus (klō' nus). A rapid series of muscular contractions and relaxations.

clostridium (klos trid' i um). A genus of bacteria that includes the causative agents of tetanus and botulism.

clotting time. The time it takes for blood to clot.

coagulase (kō ag' ū lās). The enzyme that causes the clotting of plasma.

coagulum (kō ag' ū lum). A clotted mass.

coalesce (kō a les'). To grow together into a mass.

coarctation (kō ark tā' shun). Narrowing or contraction of a blood vessel or canal.

cobalt (kō' bawlt). A metallic element.

cocaine (kō kān). A narcotic alkaloid used as a surface anesthetic. It can induce addiction.

coccus (kok' us). A spherical-shaped bacterium.

codeine (kō dēn). An opium alkaloid with analgesic properties.

coliform (kō li form). Any one of a number of bacteria found in fecal matter, which resemble Escherichia coli.

collagen (kol' a jen). An albuminous substance found in connective tissue and bone.

colloid (kol' oid). A glue-like substance that cannot diffuse through an animal membrane.

coma (kō' ma). A state of complete prolonged unconsciousness.

comedo (kom' ē do). A blackhead plugging a sebacious gland in the skin.

compazine (kom' pa zēn). A sedative, antiemetic drug.

complement (kom' plĕ ment). A constituent of plasma that is imported in immunity mechanisms.

composite resin (kom poz' it rez' in). A white filling material used primarily to restore anterior teeth.

compos mentis (kom' pōs men' tis). Of sound mind.

compress (kom' pres). A wet cloth dressing.

concretion (kon krē' shun). A hard deposit.

concussion (kon kush' un). A jarring condition of the brain caused by a blow or fall.

condenser (kon den' ser). Instrument used to pack amalgam in a cavity preparation.

condyle (kon' dil). The cylindrical process of the mandible that fits in the socket of the tempero-mandibular joint.

condyloma (kon di lo' ma). Wart-like tumors of the skin.

congential (kon jen' it al). A condition or abnormality present from birth or before.

congestion (kon je' shun). Excess blood in a given area.

contagion (kon tāg' un). Transfer of disease from person to person.

contracture (kon trak tūr). Shortening of scar tissue or muscle leading to deformity of the involved tissue.

contusion (kon tū' zhun). Minor bleeding into tissue without the skin being broken.

convolutions (kon vō lū' shunz). Coils or folds like those on the surface of the brain or the lining of the small intestine.

convulsions (kon vul' shunz). Involuntary muscle contractions by abnormal stimulation of the cerebum.

Cooley's anemia (kool' ēz anē mi a). A hemoglobin abnormality which is genetically transmitted.

copper band (kop' er band). Tube used in taking an impression of a single tooth; it is placed around the tooth being worked on.

cord. A string-like structure.

core (kŏr) The central portion. In dentistry, a "post and core" usually refers to the buildup of a prepared root canal prior to placement of a cast crown in gold, amalgam or composite.

coronary (kor' ōn a ri). Referring to the heart.

cor pulmonale (kor pul mon a' le). A heart disease that is secondary to lung disease.

corpuscle (kōr' pus l). A microscopic mass of protoplasm. Commonly refers to the blood cells, which are either red (containing hemoglobin) or white.

cortex (kor' teks). The outer layer of an organ just beneath its capsule.

corticoid (kor' ti koid). The name for the groups of natural hormone produced in the adrenal cortex. Also refers to synthetic drugs with similar actions.

corticosteroids (kor ti kō stēr' oids). Steroid hormones produced by the adrenal cortex.

cortisone (kor' ti zōn). A chief hormone of the adrenal glands used for its anti-inflammatory properties.

coryza (kor ī' za). Head cold.

coumadin (koo' ma din). A dicoumarol derivative used for its anticoagulant properties.

Coxsachie viruses (koks ak' ē vī' rus ez). One of the three groups of enteroviruses.

C.P.R. Cardiopulmonary resucitation. Emergency treatment for a person assumed to be suffering a heart attack; consists of artificial respiration and artificial circulation of the blood.

cranioplasty (krā ni o plas' ti). Surgical repair of a skull defect.

craniosynostosis (krā' ni ō sin os tō' sis). Premature calcification of the skull bones, causing facial deformities.

craniotomy (krā ni ot' ōm i). Surgical opening of the skull.

cranium (krā ni um). The top part of the skull that encloses the brain.

creatine (krē' at in). A derivative of protein found in muscle.

creatinine (krē at' in ēn). A by-product of protein metabolism found in normal urine

crepitation (krep i tā' shun). A crackling, grating sound found in bone fracture, joint disease and tissue disease.

cricoid (krī' koid). A ring-shaped cartilage forming the lower part of the larynx.

cross bite (kros bīt) Refers to an abnormal overlap of teeth.

crown (kroun). The crown of the tooth is the visible part. It consists of the pulp (blood vessels and nerves) inside the pulp chamber. This is covered by dentin and then enamel. The shape of the crown varies, depending on the type of tooth. There is a specific type of restoration referred to as a "crown," which uses metal or porcelain to cover a prepared tooth. A toothlike cap, which has been fitted to the tooth is cemented to it.

cryoanalgesia (krī ō an al jē' zi a). Pain relief accomplished by use of intense cold.

238

cryogenic (krī ō jen' ik). Caused by low temperature.

cryptogenic (krip tō jen' ik). Of unknown or obscure cause.

culture (kul' tūr). Growing of microorganisms on artificial media.

cumulative action (kū' mū lā tiv ak' shun). Repeated doses of slowly excreted drugs cause an increased action which may be toxic (e.g. barbiturates, digitalis, etc.).

curettage (kū ret' azh). The scraping of tissue from a body cavity. In dentistry, this refers to the removal of calculus from the root surface of the teeth and from the socket of an extracted tooth.

curette (kū ret'). A spoon- or loop-shaped instrument with sharp cutting edges, used to perform gingival curettage. "Scaling" usually refers to the removal of calculus from the visible tooth structure; "curettage" from below the gum and of tissue from the superfical layer of the socket. However, the term "scaler" or "curette" is often used interchangeably.

Cushingoid (Koosh' ing oid). The moon-faced, swollen appearance typical of elevated levels of corticosteroids.

cusp (kusp). An incline on the surface of each tooth that guides the teeth when they intermesh.

cuspid (kus' pid). Also known as the eye teeth or canines, the bony architecture of the face is shaped by the alveola bone of this tooth.

cutaneous (kū tā ni us). Pertaining to the skin.

cuticle (kū tik l). The outer dead-cell layer of the skin.

cyanosis (sī an ō' sis). A bluish coloration usually of the skin, nails and lips due to a lack of oxygen.

cyclopropane (sī' klō prō' pān). An anesthetic gas that is very inflammable.

cyclothymia (sī klō thī mi a). Recurrent cycles of depression and elation found in mild manic-depressive psychosis.

cyst (sist). A fluid-filled or semisolid membranous sac.

Cysteine (sis' tī ēn). A sulfur containing amino acid.

cytology (sī tol' ō ji). The microscopic study of the body cells.

cytolysis (sī tol' i sis). Disintegration and destruction of cells.

239

cytoplasm (sī' tō plazm). The protoplasm of the cell other than the nucleus.

cytotoxic (sī tō toks' ik). Any drug that destroys cells.

dactylology (dak' ti lol' o ji). A method of communication with deaf and dumb people by means of finger signs.

Dakin's solution (dāk' ins sol ū' shun). Sodium hypochlorite solution used for wound dressing and irrigation.

Darvon (dar' von). Dextroproporyphine; an analgesic.

debridement (dă brēd' ment). Thorough surgical cleaning of a wound by removal of all injured tissue and foreign material.

Decadron (dek' a drŏn). Dexamethasone—a potent anti-inflammatory steriod.

decalcification (dē kal si fik ā' shun). Loss of mineral salts from teeth or bones, such as that occuring in dental caries.

decerebrate (dē sér' ē brāt). A state of profound unconsciousness due to loss of cerebral function.

deciduous teeth (dē sid' ū us tēth). Primary teeth—often times misnomered as "baby teeth." First and second primary molars are replaced by permanent first and second bicuspids. There are 10 to 20 primary teeth in each jaw.

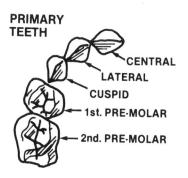

PRIMARY TEETH

CENTRAL

LATERAL

CUSPID

1st. PRE-MOLAR

2nd. PRE-MOLAR

Declomycin (dek lō mī' sin). Demethylchortetracycline; an antibiotic.

decortication (de kort ik a' shun). Removing an organ or structure by surgical means.

240

decubitus (de kū' bi tus). The lying-down position.

decussation (dē ku sā' shun). An intersection of nerve fibers past their point of origin.

degeneration (dē jen' er ā' shun). The deterioration of a tissue.

deglutition (dē gloo tish' un). The act of swallowing.

dehiscence (de his' ens). The bursting open of a tissue or organ; in dentistry, refers to an abnormal opening in bone that is commonly found in the periapical area. A dehiscence may cause exacerbation of a periodontal condition.

dehydration (dē hīd rā' shun). The loss of tissue fluids from the body with inadequate replacement.

dementia (dē men' shi á). Deterioration of mental faculties due to organic causes.

Demerol (děm' er ōl). Meperidine hydrochloride. A synthetic analgesic agent to control pain.

demulcent (dē mul' sent). A thick, soothing liquid, used on irritated mucous membranes.

demyelinization (dē mī el in īz a' shun). The breakdown and loss of the myelin sheaths that cover nerve fibers. Found especially in multiple sclerosis.

denervation (dē ner vā' shun). The cutting of a nerve supply, usually by incision.

dens in dente (denz in dentē). Developmental abnormality characterized by an enamel-lined invagination in a tooth.

dentifrice (den' ti fris). Substance used to clean teeth.

dentin (den' tin). A hard, yellowish substance that surrounds the pulp, making up most of a tooth. It is harder than bone, and consists mostly of mineral salts and water, but has some living cells. The dentin is covered by enamel above the gum, and cementum, which anchors the tooth in the socket.

dentition (den ti' shun). The naturally occurring primary and adult teeth in a patient.

denture (den' chūr). A prosthetic appliance that replaces the missing teeth. A partial denture may use the remaining teeth as support and have a cast-metal framework; a full (or complete) denture is usually all acrylic.

dermatitis (dér ma tī' tis). Skin inflammation.

dermatology (dér mat ol' ō ji). The branch of medicine that deals with the skin, its structure, function and diseases.

dermatosis (dér mat ōs' is). Skin disease.

desensitization (dē sen si tiz a' shun). The elimination of an acquired sensitivity to an external agent like a drug or plant materials.

detoxification (dē toks if a kā' shun). The removal of poisonous properties from a substance.

detritus (dē trī tus). Waste materials caused by the breaking-off from a mass.

Dexedrine (deks' e drēn). Dextroamphetamine; a stimulant of the central nervous system.

dextrose (deks' trōs). A soluble carbohydrate used in intravenous infusions; also called *glucose*.

diabetes (dī a bē' tez). A disease that causes impaired utilization of sugar in the body. Sugar appears in the urine and there is a greatly increased amount of urine.

diabetogenic (dī a bē tō jen' ik). Producing diabetes.

Diabinase (dī ab in ās). Chlorpropamide; an antidiabetic drug.

diagnosis (dī ag nō' sis). The process of differentiating one disease from another.

diagnostic model (dī ag nos' tik mod l). Plaster model of patient's mouth used for diagnostic purposes.

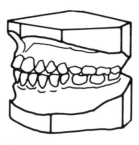

DIAGNOSTIC MODELS

diarthrosis (dī ar thrō' sis). A fluid-lubricated, freely movable joint, like the temporomandibular joint.

diastema (dī a stē' ma). Any space between teeth.

diastole (dī as' tō li). The relaxation period of the cardiac cycle.

diathermy (dī' a ther mi). The process of passing a high-frequency electric current through tissue to produce heat.

diazepam (dī az' ī pam). A sedative tranqulizer used in the treatment of psychiatric disorders like anxiety and depression.

dicumerol (dī koo' mer ol). A drug used orally as an anti-coagulant.

differential blood count (dif er en shal blud kount). The tabulation of the relative number of white cells in the blood. The normal adult count is polys, 65-70 percent; lymphocytes, 20-25 percent; monocytes, 5 percent; eosinophiles, 1-3 percent; basophils, 0.5 percent.

digestion (dī jest' chun). The conversion of food into absorbable matter.

digitalis (dij i tal' is). A drug derived from foxglove used to treat congestive heart failure and atrial fibrillation.

Digitoxin (dij it oks' in). A derivative of digitalis.

Digoxin (dij oks' in). A derivative of digitalis.

dihydrocodeine tartrate (dī hī drō ko' dēn tar' trāt). An analgesic used for treating cough and upper respiratory infections. It is nonhabit forming.

dilaceration (dī' las er ā' shun). Curvature of the root of a tooth, often causing difficulty in removal.

Dilantin (dī lan' tin). Diphenylhydantoin. A synthetic anticonvulsant used in treatment of epilepsy.

dilate (dī late). To enlarge.

dilatation (dī la tā' shun). The act of making larger by stretching or use of medication.

Dilaudid (dī law' did). Dihydromorphinone. A highly effective analgesic of the narcotic family.

diphtheria (dif thē' ri a). A highly infectious disease affecting mucous membranes usually of the upper respiratory tract.

diplopia (dip lō' pi a). Double vision.

disarticulation (dis ar tik ū lā' shun). Amputation of a bone at a joint.

disclosing agent (dis clō zing a jent). Chemical used to stain plaque on the teeth to help a patient more effectively clean his or her teeth.

dislocation (dis lō kā' shun). A displacement of bones or organs that are normally in apposition; in dentistry, this refers to the strutures that make up the temperomandibular joint.

distal (dis' tal). Descriptive term for that part of a tooth or anatomic structure away from the front.

diuretic (dī úrĕt' ik). A substance that increases urine flow.

Diuril (dī' u ril). Chlorothiazide; a diuretic.

DNA. Deoxyribonucleic acid.

DOCA. Desoxycorticosterone.

dopamine (dōp' a mĭn). A drug that is useful in treating cardiac shock and hypotension. Also used in treating Parkinsonism.

Down's Syndrome (dounz sin drōm). A condition of congenital mental retardation that includes the presence of mongoloid facial features.

doxycycline (doks ĕ sī' klin). A rapidly excreted tetracycline.

DPT. A combined vaccine which provides immunity against diphteria, pertussis and tetanus.

dressing (dres' ing). Any material used to cover a wound.

dry socket (drī sok' et). A complication following extraction of a tooth, caused by the accidental dislodgement of the organizing blood clot. Characterized by pain and necrosis of alveolar bone.

duct (dukt). A tubelike, narrow channel.

dysarthria (dis ar thria). Stammering.

dysarthrosis (dis ar thrō' sis). A joint condition that hinders movement.

dyscrasia (dis krā zhia). An abnormal condition that is a result of toxic substances in the blood.

dysfunction (dis fungk' shun). Abnormal functioning of an organ or structure.

dysorexia (dis o reks' i á). Abnormal appetite.

dyspepsia (dĭs pep' si a). Indigestion.

dysphagia (dis fā' ji a). Difficulty in swallowing.

dysplasia (dis plāz' i á). Presence of abnormal tissue.

dyspnea (disp' nē a). Difficult breathing.

dystrophy (dis' trō fǐ). Defective nutrition that can lead to a variety of disorders of body organs or systems.

ecchondroma (ek kon drō' má). A benign tumor arising from cartilage, and protruding out from its surface.

ecchymosis (ek i mō' sis). Subcutaneous bleeding into the tissues.

ectopia (ek tō' pi á). Malposition of a structure or organ.

eczema (ek' zē má). A form of dermatitis usually characterized by vesicle formation and scaliness.

edema (e dē' má). Abnormal fluid infiltration of tissues.

edentulous (ē dent' ū lus). Lacking teeth.

efferent (ĕf fer ent). Carrying away from a central point.

effusion (e fū' zhun). Infiltration of fluid into the tissues and organ cavities.

Elavil (el' a vil). Amitriptyline. An antidepressant drug.

electrodessication (ē lek trō des i kā' shun). Surgical drying and removal of tissue using electrodes.

electromyography (e lek trō mǐ og' ra fi). Recording of electric currents from muscle tissue.

electrosurgery (ē lek' trō sur' je ri). Cauterization by an electric current.

elevator (el e vā ter). Instrument used between socket and tooth in oral surgery to help loosen a tooth prior to forceps extraction.

elixir (e lik' sèr). A sweetened solution of a drug that contains alcohol.

embolism (em' bō lism). Plugging of a blood vessel by solid materials like blood clots or fat particles, or by air bubbles.

emesis (em' i sis). The act of vomiting.

emollient (ē mōl' i ent). A softening agent used on skin or mucosa.

emphysema (em fi sē' ma). Distension of tissue by gas. In pulmonary emphysema, it can either be localized or generalized throughout the entire lung.

empyema (em pī ē' ma). A concentration of pus in a body organ or space.

emulsion (ē mul' shun). A liquid containing suspended particles of fat or oil.

enamel (en am' el). Enamel overlies the dentin in the crown of the tooth, forming the outermost covering of the crown. It is the hardest substance in the body. Enamel is white, but transparent. Teeth appear yellowish because the dentin, below the enamel, shows through. As the tooth wears away, the dentin becomes exposed, causing a sensitivity to hot and cold foods and particularly liquids.

endarterectomy (end árt e rek' to mi). Surgical removal of a atherosclerotic plug from an artery.

endemic (en dem' ik). Locally recurring.

endocarditis (en dō kar dī' tis). Inflammation of the membrane that lines the inside of the heart.

endocardium (eń dō kar di um). The inner-lining membrane of the heart.

endogenous (en doj' e nus). Occurring inside the body.

endophlebitis (en' dō fle bī' tis). Inflammation of the inner lining of a vein.

endoscope (en' dō skōp). An instrument used to visualize and examine the internal organs or cavities of the body.

endotoxin (en dō tok' sin). A poisonous bacterial product that occurs inside the cell.

enterovirus (en ter ō vī' rus). A virus that enters the body via the digestive tract.

enucleation (e nu klē ā' shun). The removal of an entire organ or mass.

enzyme (en' zīm). A soluble protein produced by living cells, which aids in metabolism.

eosinophil (ē ō sin' ō fil). A specific type of white blood cell that is stained by the dye eosin.

ephedrine (ĕ fĕd' rin). A vasoconstricting drug used in treating asthma and hay fever.

epidemiology (ep i dēm ī ol' ō ji). The study of the occurence and distribution of disease.

epidermis (ep i der' mis). The outside layer of the skin.

epidural (ep i dū ral). External to the outer membrane of the brain or spinal cord.

epiglottis (ep i glot' is). A thin cartilage structure behind the tongue that aids in the act of swallowing.

epilepsy (eṕ i lep' si). A series of disorders caused by abnormal electrical activity of the brain. It is marked by fits and/or fainting.

epinephrine (ep i nef' rin). Adrenalin.

epiphysis (ē pif' i sis). That part of bones, especially the long ones, which contain the growing areas.

epistaxis (ep i stak' sis). Nosebleed.

epithelioma (ep i thēl i ō' ma). A malignant tumor of epithelial tissue.

epithelium (ep i thē li um). The surface cell layer covering skin, mucous and serous surfaces.

epulis (e pū lis). A benign gum tumor.

Equanil (e' kwan il). Meprobamate or Miltown; a tranquilizer.

ergometry (er gom' et ri). The measurement of the work output of muscle.

erosion (ē rō' zhun). Process of wearing away of tooth structure, often by too-vigorous brushing or using a too-hard bristled brush.

ergosterol (èr gos' tér ōl). A naturally occuring previtamin that is converted to vitamin D by sunlight exposure.

eructation (e ruk tā' shun). Belching.

erysipelas (er i sip' e las). An acute streptococcal infection of the skin and subcutaneous structures.

erythema (e ri thē' ma). Skin reddening.

erythrocyte (e rith' rō sīt). Red blood cell.

erythrocythemia (ē rith rō si thē' mi a). Increased production of red blood cells.

erythrocytopenia (ē rith rō sī tō pē' ni a). Deficient numbers of red blood cells.

erythromycin (ē rith rō mī' sin). An orally administered antibiotic with actions similar to penicillin.

escharotic (es ka rot ik). Any agent that produces a sloughing of tissue.

esophagectomy (ē sof' a jek' to mē). Surgical removal of all or part of the esophagus.

esophagitis (ē sof a jī' tis). Inflammation of the esophagus.

esophagus (ē sof' a gus). The muscular canal that connects the stomach to the pharynx. Also called the gullet.

esthetics (es thet' iks). The techniques used to match the form and color of the natural teeth most closely when placing restorations or prostheses.

ethmoid (eth' moid). The spongy bone forming part of the nose.

ethyl chloride (eth' il klor' īd). An anesthetic that can be for either local or general administration.

etiology (ē ti ol' o ji). The causes of disease.

euphoria (ū for' ē a). An exaggerated feeling of well-being.

eustachian (ū stā' ki an). A partly bony canal connecting the inner ear with the pharynx.

Evipan (ev' i pan). Hexobarbital; a short-acting barbiturate.

evulsion (ē vul' shun). Tearing away of a structure by force.

exacerbation (eks as er bā' shun). An increase in severity.

exanthema (eks an thē ma). A skin eruption.

excavator (eks' ka vā ter). Instrument used to remove decay from a tooth; often called a "spoon" excavation.

excresence (eks kres' ens). An abnormal outgrowth of the tissues.

exfoliation (eks fō li ā' shun). The peeling off of tissues, by layers. Also the normal loss of the primary teeth.

exocrine (eks' o krin). Glands that secrete via a duct.

exodontics (eks ō don' tiks). Surgical removal of the teeth.

exogenous (eks oj' ē nus). Originating externally.

exostosis (eks os tō' sis). A bony outgrowth.

exsanguination (eks sang gwi nā' shun). The act of making bloodless.

extensor (eks ten' sor). A muscle that straightens a limb or part of the body.

extradural (eks tra dūr' al). Outside of the dura mater (the membrane which covers the brain).

extravasation (eks trav a sā' shun). The leaking of fluid from its normal enclosure into the surrounding tissues.

extrinsic (eks trin' sik). Originating from the outside.

extroversion (eks tro ver' shun). Concentration on outside activities rather than on one's inner self.

extrusion (eks' trōō zhun). Super eruption of a tooth when the opposing tooth is lost.

exudate (eks' ū dāt). Fluid that leaks out.

exudation (eks' ū dā' shun). The leaking of fluid through capillary walls.

Facebow (fās bō). Instrument used in prosthodontics to transfer a patient's bite to stone models.

Fahrenheit (far' en hīt). A temperature scale in which the boiling point is 212°, and the freezing point is 32°.

fascia (fash' i à). The fibrous sheath that connects the skin to the underlying tissues. It also covers and contains muscles.

fauces (fau' sēz). The opening between the mouth and the pharynx.

F.D.A. The federal "Food and Drug Administration."

febrile (feb' rīl). The presence of fever.

fenestration (fen es trā' shun). The surgical creation of an opening in the inner ear to treat certain types of deafness.

fetor (fē' tor). A strong, offensive odor.

fibrin (fī' brin). A protein formed by clotting blood.

fibroblast (fi' brō blast). A cell that helps produce connective tissue.

fibroma (fī brō' mȧ). A benign tumor consisting of fibrous tissue.

fibrosis (fīb brō' sis). The development of excess fibrous tissue in a structure that normally does not contain it.

fissure (fish' er). A pit or chasm in a tooth that renders it more susceptible to decay.

fistula (fis' tū lȧ). An abnormal opening between two cavities of surfaces of the body.

fixed bridge (fikst brij). Nonremovable replacement for missing teeth; cemented permanently.

FIXED BRIDGE

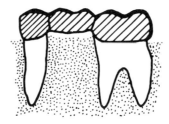

flap (flap). A procedure that consists of incising and reflecting the gums for access to the root and alveolar bone.

flexor (flek' sor). A muscle that, when it contracts, bends a body part.

flexure (flek' sher). A bend in a body structure.

flouridation (floor' id ā shun). Addition of flourine to water, usually as an anticaries measure.

fluoroscopy (floor' os' kō pi). The use of a flourescent screen for X-ray examination.

follicle (fol' i kl). A small tubular sac or gland.

fontanel (fon ta nel'). A thin membranous space between the bones of the skull.

foramen (for ā' men). A hole or opening, generally in a bone.

forceps (for' seps). Surgical instruments used for grasping or holding.

forensic medicine (fo ren' sik med' i sin). The use of medical information in questions of law.

formulary (for' mū ler i). A list of formulas.

fossa (fos' a). A depression or groove.

fracture (frak' tūr). A break in the continuity of a bone.

frenum (frē' num). A piece of tissue which acts to limit the movement of a muscle.

friable (frī ab l). Easily breakable into small pieces.

fulguration (ful gū rā' shun). The use of electrical current or diathery to destroy tissue.

full-cast gold crown. (fŏŏl kast kroun). A replacement for the entire coronal portion of a tooth. Usually used when a tooth is shattered or carious beyond repair by any other means; not a gold "cap."

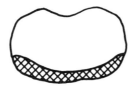

**FULL CAST GOLD
CROWN**

full denture (fŏŏl den' tūr). Prosthetic replacement for all upper or lower teeth. Term often used by patients is "plate."

fulminant (ful' mi nant). Developing and ending with great severity and intensity.

fungicide (fun' ji sīd). A fungus-destroying agent.

gag reflex (gag rē' fleks). Uncontrollable retching that may be produced when the soft palate is touched. Can be a problem when taking impressions.

gamma globulin (gam' ma glob' ū lin). A protein that is produced by the body, and employed in its immune responses.

ganglion (gang' glē on). A concentrated mass of nerve tissue forming a center that receives and sends out nerve fibers.

gangrene (gang' grēn). Tissue death of a part of the body.

gelfoam (jel fōm). An absorbable gelatin used to pack the socket of an extracted tooth.

gemination (jem' i nā' shun). Developmental deformity of a tooth in which the crown attempts to divide.

gene (jēn). A chromosomal factor that transmits hereditary characteristics.

generic (je ner' ik). Referring to drugs, it is the distinctive identifying name and is not protected by a trademark.

genetics (jē net' iks). The study of heredity.

genial tubercles (je nī' al tu' ber klz). Bony prominences of the chin.

geriatrics (jer i at' riks). The branch of medicine dealing with old age and its diseases.

gerontology (jer on tol' ō ji). The science dealing with aging.

gingiva (jin ji' va). The gums, or soft tissue around the teeth.

gingivectomy (jin ji vek' tō mi). The surgical removal of part of the gums.

gingivitis (jin ji vī' tis). Inflammation of the gums.

giromatic (jī' rō ma tic). Type of drill used to instrument a root canal.

gland (glănd). An organ that produces a secretion.

glaucoma (glŏ kō' ma). An eye disease in which the intraocular pressure is elevated.

glenoid fossa (glē' noid fos' a). Socket into which the temperomandibular joint rests.

glioma (glī ō' mȧ). A malignant growth.

glossa (glos' a). The tongue.

glossopharyngeal (glos ō fa rin jē al). Referring to the tongue and pharynx.

glottis (glot' is). The part of the larynx that helps create vocal sounds.

glucose (glŏŏ' kōs). Dextrose. It is the form in which carbohydrates are metabolized and circulated in the blood.

glycogen (gli' kō jen). The animal starch in which form glucose is stored in the body.

goiter (goi' ter). An enlargement of the thyroid gland.

gold foil (gōld foil). Type of direct gold filling material.

gonococcus (gon ō kok' us). The bacteria that causes gonorrhea.

gonorrhea (gon o rē' å). An infectious venereal disease in adults. Children are accidentally infected.

gout (gowt). A painful metabolic disorder that is characterized by deposits of sodium biurate in cartilage throughout the body, and uric acid in the urine.

Gow-Gates technique. (gow gātz). An injection that anesthetizes half of the face by numbing the trigeminal (Gasserian) ganglion.

gran mal (gran' mal). The major form of epilepsy, characterized by unconsciousness and convulsions.

granuloma (gran ū lō' må). A benign tumor containing granulation tissue.

ground substance (ground sub' stans). Intercellular material in most soft tissue.

gums (gumz). Firm, pink flesh around the roots of the teeth. When the gums and the bones surrounding the teeth become diseased, it is called *periodontitis*.

gumma (gum' å). A characteristic localized area of vascular-granulated tissue found in the later stage of syphlis. It may be found in or around the oral cavity.

gutta percha (gut'a per cha). Material used to fill root canals or for temporary fillings.

habit (hab' it). Behavior that is repeated often.

hallucinogens (ha lū' si nō jens). Chemicals that produce false perceptions without true physical cause.

Hansen's disease (han senz di zēz). Leprosy.

hare lip. (har lip). A congenital deformity of the lip and/or palate due to incomplete fusion of the embryonic processes that may leave an opening between the nasal and oral cavities.

Haversian systems (hǎ ver si'an sis' temz). Series of nutrient canals in bone.

Hawley appliance (haw lē a plī ans). A device fabricated to retain the desired effects of tooth movement following orthodontics. It consists of an acrylic base and wrought wire clasps that must be worn after removal of the braces.

helix (hē' liks). The outer edge of the external ear.

helminthiasis (hel min thī' a sis). The syndrome caused by infestation with worms.

hemangioma (he man ji ō' mȧ). A blood-vessel malformation that can occur in any area of the body.

hematemesis (hē ma tem' e sis). Vomiting blood.

hematuria (hē ma tū' ri ȧ). Blood in the urine.

hemiglossectomy (hem i glos ek' tō mi). Removal of approximately half the tongue.

hemiplegia (hem i plē' ji ȧ). Paralysis affecting half of the body.

hemoglobin (hē mō glō' bin). The iron containing pigment in red blood corpuscles. It combines with oxygen and then releases it in the tissues.

hemophilia (hē mō fil' i a). An inherited bleeding disease usually only affecting males.

hemoptysis (hē mop' ti sis). Coughing up blood.

hemorrhage (hem o rij). The escape of blood from a blood vessel.

hemostasis (hē mō stā' sis). The stoppage of bleeding.

heparin (hep' ar in). A substance found in liver and lung tissue that inhibits blood clotting when injected.

hepatitis (hep a tī' tis). Inflammation of the liver caused by viral infection.

herpes (her' pēz). A vesicular eruption due to viral infection. Oral herpes is extrememly common and is often called "cold sores" or canker sores.

hiatus (hī ā' tus). An opening.

hilum (hī' lum). A groove or depression on the surface of an organ where other structures enter or leave.

hirsute (hėr' sūt). Hairy.

histamine (his' ta mēn). A chemical that appears normally in body tissue. It affects muscle, capillary and gastric function, and is released during allergic or inflammatory attacks.

histology (his tol'' ō ji). The science of microscopic study of tissues.

home care. Patient's oral hygiene.

homograft (hō' mō graft). A tissue or organ transplant from one individual to another of the same species.

homologous (ho mol' ō gus). Similar in structure and origin.

hormone (hor' mōn). Chemicals secreted by an endocrine gland. It is transported by the blood stream to regulate tissue and organ function throughout the body.

host (hōst). The structure that parasites live on.

hyaline (hī a lēn). Glasslike; describes a type of membrane.

hydrocephalus (hī drō sef' a lus). An excessive amount of fluid inside the skull caused by defective cerebrospinal fluid circulation, causing pronounced swelling of the head.

hydrocolloid (hī drō kol' oid). Reversible-impression material that requires flowing water to solidify.

hydrocortisone (hī drō kor' ti zōn). An adrenal cortical steroid.

hydrolysis (hī drol' i sis). The splitting of a substance into simpler substances by the addition of water.

hydroxyapatite (hī droks i a pa tīt). Mineral whose crystals, embedded in an inorganic matrix, constitute enamel.

hygienist (hī jēn ist). Dental auxiliary who is responsible for cleaning the teeth and the education of patients about periodontal care.

hyoid (hī' oid). A bone in the throat.

hyperalgesia (hī pėr al jēz' i a). Abnormally increased pain sensitivity.

hyperbaric (hī pėr bar' ik). Exposed to greater pressure, specific gravity or weight than normal. Hyperbaric chambers are used to treat decompression sickness ("the bends").

hyperemia (hī pėr ē' mi a). Excessive blood in an area.

hyperesthesia (hī pėr es thē' zhi a). Excessive sensitivity of a part.

hyperglycemia (hī pėr glī' sē' mi a). Abnormally increased blood sugar.

hyperinsulinism (hī pėr in' sūl in izm). Excessive insulin in the blood leading to lowered blood sugar levels and loss of consciousness.

hypermotility (hī pėr mō til' i ti). An increase in movement.

hyperplasia (hī pėr plā' zhi ȧ). Excessive cell formation.

hypertension (hī pėr ten' shun). Abnormally high blood pressure.

hypertonic (hī pėr ton' ik). Having a greater osmotic pressure than physiological body fluid.

hypertrophy (hī pėr' trō fi). Abnormal increase in tissue or organ size.

hyperventilation (hī pėr ven til ā' shun). Deep, rapid breathing; hyperpnea.

hypochondria (hī pō kon' dri a). Abnormally great anxiety about one's health.

hypoglycemia (hī pō glī sē' mi a). Lowered blood sugar.

hypoplasia (hī pō plā' zhi a). Defective tissue development.

hypotension (hī pō ten' shun). Low blood pressure.

hypothermia (hī pō thėr' mi a). Abnormally low body temperature.

hypoxia (hī pok' si a). Lowered amount of oxygen in the tissues.

hysterectomy (his ter ek' tō mi). Surgical excision of the uterus.

hysteria (his tē' ri a). A neurotic disorder that exhibits a variety of physical symptoms. It is usually a result of mental conflict.

iatrogenic (ī at rō jen' ik). A secondary medical disorder resulting from treatment of a previous condition.

icterus (ik' ter us). Jaundice. *Icterus gravis* is acute liver necrosis.

idiopathy (id i op' a thi). A disease state whose cause is unknown.

idiosyncrasy (id iō sing' kra si). An unusual reaction to a drug, either by swallowing, contact, injection or inhalation.

immunity (i mū ni ti). A condition of resistance to infection.

256

Active immunity is acquired by actual contact, or infection. *Passive immunity* is by contact with the antibodies of the disease through maternal milk, via the placenta, or by injection or injestion of the immune sera.

immunization (im ū ni zā shun). The process of increasing antibodies for specifc disease within the body.

immunosuppressive (i mūn ō sup res' iv). A condition or substance that inhibits the immune response of the body to a foreign agent.

impacted (im pak' ted). Abnormally wedged or immovable. In dentistry, this refers to teeth that are prevented from erupting normally. Often, these are third molars.

impaction (im pak' shun). A trapped, unable to erupt, tooth; usually a third molar or a cuspid.

IMPACTION

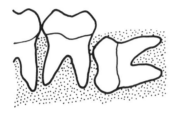

implant (im plant'). Any artificial substance placed within the body. Dental implants are used to provide a stable structure for crowns or bridges.

implantologist (im' plant ol ō gist). Specialist in replacing lost dental structures by use of devices placed within the bone or gum to which artificial teeth are attached.

impression (im prĕsh' un). A negative likeness in dentistry. With plaster and other similar materials, an impression can be taken of an entire arch or a single tooth, depending on the purpose of the impression.

incision (in sizh' un). Any perforation of soft tissue.

incision and drainage (in sizh' un and drān' ij). Technique for evacuating pus from an infection.

incisors (in sī' zerz). The front teeth that function to cut food. They are the chief biting teeth, with sharp cutting edges. Incisors have one root.

incompatibility (in kom pat' i bil' i ti). 1. A reaction that occurs when two or more medications interact after administration, causing markedly altered effects than those desired. 2. A reaction that occurs when two blood types are mixed in transfusion causing agglutination (clotting). 3. The rejection by the body of any foreign body placed within it.

Inderal (in' der al). Propranolol; used to prevent and control cardiac arrythmias and dysrhythmias.

infant (in' fant). A child of less than one year.

infarct (in' fàrkt). An area of tissue whose immediate blood supply is blocked.

infection (in fek' shun). The invasion and successful growth of microorganisms in host tissue.

infectious mononucleosis (in fek' shus mon ō nū klē ō sis). A virally caused glandular fever.

infiltration (in fil trā' shun). Penetration into surrounding tissues. One technique used for injection of anesthesia in dentistry.

inflammation (in fla mā' shun). The reaction of living tissues to infection or injury. The cardinal signs of it are redness, pain, heat and swelling.

infusion (in fū' zhun). 1. A solution containing the active ingredient of a drug, made by pouring boiling water on it. 2. Gravity flow of fluid into the body.

inlay (in lā'). A cast restoration used to replace lost tooth structure. An inlay is surrounded by sound tooth structure but

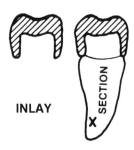

INLAY

SECTION

does not cover the cusp of a posterior tooth. When the restoration is extended to cover the cusps, the term used is onlay. Both may be fabricated directly in the mouth or on a plaster model poured from an impression.

inoculation (in ok ū lā' shun). Introduction of vaccine into the body tissue.

in situ (in sit' ū). In the correct position.

insulin (in' sū lin). A hormone manufactured in the pancreas, and secreted into the blood. It regulates carbohydrate metabolism.

integument (in teg' ū ment). A covering, usually of the skin.

interarticular (in tėr år tik' ū lar). Between joint-articulating surfaces.

interdental papillae (in ter den' tal pa pil' a). Triangular gum tissue located between teeth.

interferon (in ter fē' ron). A naturally occurring protein that can destroy viruses.

interproximal (in' ter prŏk' si mal). Referring to the areas between the teeth.

interstice (in tur' stis). A space.

interstitial (in tėr stish' al). Located in the spaces of a structure.

intolerance (in tol' er ans). Inability to react normally to certain drugs.

intra (in' tra). Prefix meaning within.

intrinsic (in trin' sik). Natural or real; inherent.

introversion (in trō ver' zhun). The turning inward of mental processes and thoughts.

intrusion (in trōō' zhun). Method of forcing a tooth deeper into it's socket, using braces and wires.

intubation (in tū bā' shun). Placement of a tube into a hollow organ, usually the larynx.

invagination (in vaj in ā' shun). Pushing inward to form a pouch.

inversion (in ver' zhun). Turning inside out.

involution (in vo lū' shun). The normal decrease in size of an organ after it completes its function.

irrigation (ir i gā' shun). Flushing of any structure with liquid.

ischemia (is kē' mi a). Lowered blood supply.

isotonic (i sō ton' ik). The same osomotic pressure as blood.

jacket crown (jak' et kroun). In prosthodontics, all porcelain coverage of a tooth, usually an anterior one.

jaundice (jawn' dis). A pathological state characterized by an increased bilirubin level in the blood. The primary sign is yellow skin.

joint (joynt). An articulation between bones.

jugular (jug' ū lar). Relating to the throat.

Kanamycin (kan a mī sin). A streptomycin-like antibiotic.

keloid (kē loid). An abnormal increase in scar tissue that may produce a deformity.

keratin (ker' a tin). A protein that is resistant to acid.

keratosis (ker a tō sis). Thickening of the outer skin layer.

kinesthesis (kin es thē' sis). Sensation of movement.

Koplik's spots (Kop liks spotz). Small white spots found in the mouth during the earliest stage of measles.

labia (lā' bi a). Lip-like folds; also synonomous with lips.

labial (lā' bi al). In dentistry, refers to the tooth surface closest to the lips.

lacrimal (lak' ri mal). Referring to tears.

lacunae (la kū na). Series of hollows in bone.

laryngeal (la rin jē al). Referring to the larynx.

laryngoscope (lar in' gō skōp). An instrument used to examine the inside of the larynx.

larynx (lar' ingks). The vocal organ located interior to and below the pharynx.

L-dopa (el dō' pa). Levodopa. A synthetic drug used in the treatment of Parkinson's disease.

lateral condensation (lat' er al kon' den sā' shun). Technique for filling a root canal.

260

lateral periodontal abcess (lat' er al per i ō don' tal ab ses). Infection of the gums located on the mucosa that may involve adjacent teeth.

lecithin (les' i thin). A fatty substance found in cell protoplasm.

lentigo (len tī' gō). A freckle.

lesion (le' zhun). Abnormal change in a body tissue.

lethal (lē' thal). Leading to death.

leucine (lū' sēn). An essential amino acid.

leukemia (lū kē' mi a). A malignant blood disease characterized by abnormal numbers or types of white blood cells.

leukocytes (lū' kō sīts). The white blood cells. They include: *polymorphonuclear, basophile, eosinophile, lymphocyte* and *monocyte.*

leukocytosis (lū kō sī tō' sis). Abnormal increase in number of white blood cells in the blood.

leukopenia (lū kō pē' ni a). Decreased number of white blood cells in the blood.

leukoplakia (lū kō plā ki' a). A whitish, thickened patch seen on mucous membrane of mouth or genitals.

librium (lib rē um). Trade name for one of the major tranquilizers.

lichen (lī' ken). A collection of small, raised skin lesions.

Lidocaine (līd' ō kān). A local anesthetic. Commonly, but incorrectly, labelled as "novocaine."

ligament (lig' a ment). A strong, fibrous band of tissue that supports or binds together organs or bones.

ligate (lī' gāt). To bind or tie up.

ligature (lig' a tūr). The material used to sew or tie up tissue or vessels.

Lincocin (lin' kō sin). Lincomycin; an antibiotic.

lingua (lin' gwa). The tongue.

lingual (ling' gwal). Surface of tooth facing the tongue.

lipemia (lĭ pē' mi a). Increased fats in the blood.

lipoid (li' poid). Resembling fats.

lipoma (lip ō' ma). A benign fatty tumor.

liquefaction necrosis (li kwa fak' shun nek rō' sis). A type of cellular death.

lithiasis (lith ī a sis). Formation of calculi or stone in the body.

liver (liv' er). The largest organ in the body. It lies in the upper-right section of the abdomen, and secretes bile, produces and stores glycogen, and helps regulate fat and protein metabolism.

lobe (lōb). A round part of an organ, usually separated from the rest of it by a fissure or septum.

long buccal (long buk' al). Type of injection given to anesthetize the molars of the lower jaw when administered with a mandibular-block injection.

lorazepam (lor az' ē pam). A tranquilizer.

loupe (loop). A magnifying lens.

lues (lū' ēz). Syphilis.

lumen (loo' men). The interior of a tubular structure.

lupus (loo' pus). A nodular skin disease.

luxation (luks a' shun). A dislocation.

lymph (limf). The transparent fluid carried by the lymphatic vessels.

lymphadenitis (lim fad ē nī' tis). Inflammation of one or more of the lymph nodes.

lymphangioma (lim fan ji ō' ma). A benign tumor of the lymph vessels.

lymphocyte (lim' fō sīt). One type of white blood cell.

lymphoma (lim fō' ma) A benign tumor or lymphatic tissue.

lysine (lī' sēn). An essential amino acid.

macrocephalous (mak rō sef' a lus). Excessive development of the head caused by genetic or disease processes.

macrocyte (mak' rō sīt). A large red blood cell, seen in the blood in some anemias.

macroglossia (mak rō glos' i a). Abnormally large tongue.

macrophage (mak' rō fāj). A large phagocytic blood cell, found in connective tissue.

maintainer (mān tān' er). Device used to retain space for the erupting dentition, often following premature loss of primary teeth.

malacia (ma lā' shia). Softening of a body structure.

malignant (ma lig' nant). Tending to cause death, as a disease or tumor.

malingering (ma ling' ger ing). Pretending illness to avoid work or an unpleasant situation.

malocclusion (mal o klōō' zhun). A faulty coming together of the upper and lower teeth. Orthodontics is the specialty that treats this problem.

malpractice (mal prak' tis). Failure of a professional person to render treatment through ignorance, carelessness or criminal intent.

mandible (man' di bl). The lower jaw bone.

mandibular (man dib' ū lar). Referring to the lower jaw.

mania (mā' ni a). A psychosis, characterized by excessive excitement and possibly violence.

marezine (măr' e zēn). A short-acting antihistamine, contraindicated in pregnancy.

marsupialization (mar sū pi al i zā' shun). A surgical procedure used in treating cystic conditions.

mastication (mas ti kā' shun). The chewing act.

mastoid (mas toid'). The nipplelike process of the temporal bone, located behind the ear.

mastoiditis (mas toid ī' tis). Inflammation of the mastoid air cells.

materia medica (mat ē' ri a med' ika) The science of drugs, their sources, actions and dosage.

mattress suture (mat' ris sū' tur). Method of stitching wounds or incisions.

matrix (mā triks). A metal or plastic band adapted to a tooth to allow condensation of amalgam or composite. It is held in place with a retainer and wedge.

maxilla (mak sil' a). The upper jaw bone.

maxillary (mak' si ler i). Referring to the upper arch.

measles (mē z lz). An acute viral disease that is highly infectious.

meatus (mē ā' tus). An open channel.

meclizine (mek' li zēn). An antihistamine.

media (mē' di a). A jelly-like substance, containing nutrients, that is used in culturing bacteria. The middle layer of a vessel.

medial (mē' di al). Referring to the middle.

Medrol (med' rōl). Methylprednisolone, an anti- inflammatory steroid.

medulla (me dul' a). The marrow-containing center of long bones. The internal, soft center of glands.

megacephalic (me ga se fal' ik). Abnormally large head.

melanin (mel' a nin). A black pigment found in the body.

melanoma (mel a nō ma). A malignant tumor arising from the pigment cells of the skin or eye.

melanosis (mel a nō sis). Dark, surface pigmentation.

membrane (mem' brān). A thin, surface covering, or lining.

menadione (men a dī' ōn). Vitamin K.

meninges (me nin jēs). The covering membrane of the brain and spinal cord.

meniscus (men nis' kus). Crescent-shaped cartilage, especially in the temperomandibular joint.

meperidine (mep er' i dēn). A synthetic analgesic used in place of morphine.

Mepivicaine (mep iv i kān). A local anesthetic.

mercurialism (měr kū' ri al izm). Mercury poisoning.

mercury (měr kū re). Element that is a component of amalgam.

mesial (mē' zi al). Description of tooth surfaces closest to the midline.

microleakage (mī krō lēk ij). Failure of a restoration due to breakdown of material at the margins.

Miltown (mil' town). Meprobamate, a mild tranquilizer.

mitosis (mī tō' sis). The common form of cell division in specialized tissue.

mitral (mī' tral). The name for the valve between the left atrium and ventricle of the heart.

mixed dentition (mikst den tish' un). State in which primary and secondary teeth are present concurrently.

mobility (mō bil' i ti). Clinical description of a tooth that is movable within its socket. Usually expressed as I, II or III (I the least mobile).

molar (mō' ler). The back teeth, used primarily for chewing, by grinding food. They normally have three to five cusps, and two to three roots.

molecule (mol' ĕ kūl). The smallest physical particle into which matter can be divided and still retain its properties.

mongolism (mong' gol izm). The condition of a congenital, mentally deficient child born with a flattened skull and narrow slanting eyes. Also called *Downs Syndrome*.

monilia (mo nil' i a). A fungus (synonym *Candida*) which may be found in the mouth, throat, vagina, intestines or on the skin.

mononucleosis (mon ō nū klē ō' sis). A condition characterized by an increase in the number of monocytes circulating in the blood.

moribund (mor' i bund). Near death.

morphine (mor' fēn). A widely used analgesic derived from opium.

morphology (mor fol' ōj i). The study of the form and structure of living organisms.

motile (mō' til). Able to move spontaneously.

mucin (mū' sin). A mixture of glandular and cellular secretions containing glycoproteins.

mucocele (mū' kō sēl). A cavity swollen with mucus.

mucoid (mū' koid). Mucous-like.

mucosa (mū kō' sa). Mucous membrane.

mucous (mū' kus). Mucus. The thick fluidic secretion of mucous glands.

multilocular (mul ti lok' ū lar). Containing many small compartments or cells.

multipara (mul ti' par a). A woman who has borne more than one baby.

mural (mur' al). Relating to the wall of an organ, cavity or vessel.

murmur (mer' mer). An abnormal sound heard on listening with a stethoscope to the heart or a major blood vessel.

muscular dystrophy (mus' kū lar dis' trō fē). A disease of unknown cause, which leads to progressive muscular deterioration.

myalgia (mī al' ji a). Muscular pain.

myasthenia (mī as thē' ni a). Muscular weakness; myasthenia gravis is a disease causing severe fatigability of voluntary muscles.

mycology (mī kol' ō ji). The study of fungi.

mycosis (mī kō' sis). A fungus-caused disease.

myelin (mī' e lin). The fatty substance that forms the sheath or cover of nerves.

mylohyoid ridge (mī lō hī' oid rij). An anatomical feature of the lower jaw, found on the posterior buccal aspect of the mandible.

myocele (mī' o sēl). A condition in which a muscle protrudes through its ruptured sheath.

myofibrosis (mī ō fi brō' sis). Excessive deposits of fibrous connective tissue in muscle, leading to impaired function.

myoma (mī ō' ma). A muscle tissue tumor.

myositis (mī ō sī' tis). Muscle inflammation.

myxedema (mik sĕ dē' ma). Clinical condition caused by hypothyroidism. The symptoms are mental and physical slowness, dry skin, swelling of the face and limbs and lowered body temperature.

myxoma (miks ō' ma). A mucoid-containing tumor of connective tissue.

myxoviruses (miks ō vī' rus ez). The term for the influenza-causing viruses.

nalorphine (nal or' fēn). An intravenously or intramuscularly injected drug that neutralizes the action of morphine and similar depressants.

Naprosyn (nap' rō sin). An anti-inflammatory drug.

narcotic (nar kot' ik). A sleep-inducing drug.

nasopharynx (nā zō far' inks). The part of the pharynx above the soft palate.

necrosis (ne krō' sis). Localized tissue death.

necrotizing ulcerative gingevitis (nek' rō tiz ing ul' cer ā tiv jin ji vit is). Trench mouth. A condition of rapid loss of alveolar bone caused by severe periodontal infection.

Nembutal (nem' bū tal). Pentobarbital; a short-acting barbiturate.

neomycin (nē ō mī' sin). An antibiotic used for skin and intestinal infections.

neonatal (nē ō nā' tal). The first month of an infant's life.

neoplasm (nē' ō plazm). A tumor.

nephrology (nef rol' o ji). The study of kidneys and associated diseases.

neural (nūr' al). Pertaining to nerves.

neuralgia (nū ral' ji a). Pain along the course of a nerve that may be of no discernable cause.

neurastenia (nū ras thē' ni a). A nervous condition characterized by fatigue, weakness, loss of initiative and hypersensitivity.

neurilemma (nū ril lem' a). The thin, outer sheath of a nerve fiber.

neuritis (nū rī' tis). Inflammation of a nerve.

neurogenic (nū rō jen' ik). Originating in nerve tissue.

neurology (nūr ol' ō ji). The branch of medicine dealing with diseases of the nervous system.

neuroplasty (nūr' ō plas ti). Surgical nerve repair.

neurosis (nū rō' sis). A psychologically caused disorder that may result from environmental stress and anxiety.

neutropenia (nū trō pē' ni a). A relative shortage of neutrophiles.

neutrophil (nū' trō fil). A type of polymorphonuclear leukocyte.

nevus (nē' vus). A congenital skin lesion including moles and birthmarks.

nitroglycerine (nīt rō glis' er in). A vasodilator used in tablet form to treat angina pectoris.

nitrous oxide (nī' trus ox' sīd). An anesthetic, used in gaseous state.

node (nōd). A lump or swelling.

nucleus (nū' klē us). The central, essential part of cells that regulates growth and reproduction.

nutrient (nū' tri ent). A substance that provides nourishment.

nystatin (nī' stat in). An antifungal antibiotic used to treat monilial infections.

N2-Sargenti (enn two sar jen' tī). A technique of preparing and filling root canals that employs a semisolid paste containing a fixative to fill the canal. Unlike traditional root canal therapy, N2 therapy can be completed in one or two visits.

obturator (ob' tū rā tor). A device that closes an opening in the body. In dentistry, these are frequently fabricated to treat a cleft palate, or following the removal of a tumor.

occipital (ok sip' i tal). Referring to the posterior part of the skull.

occlusal traumatism (o kloo' zal tro' ma tiz m). Condition where abnormal meeting of teeth causes pain or bone loss.

occlusion (ō klōō' zhun). 1. The sealing of an opening, especially blood vessels or ducts (e.g. occlusion of the coronary artery). 2. The relationship of the upper and lower teeth when the jaws are closed.

odontalgia (ō don tal' ji a). Toothache.

odontoma (ō don tō' ma). A benign tumor that contains tooth structure.

oncology (on kol' ō ji). The study of neoplasms.

open bite (ō' pin bīt). Condition where premature meeting of some teeth prevents others from meeting evenly.

opsonin (op' son in). An antibody that aids phagocytosis.

oral surgeon (ō' ral sur' jun). Specialist who diagnoses and treats diseases, injuries and defects of the jaws and associated structures.

orbit (or' bit). The bony socket that contains and protects the eyeball.

organism (or' gan izm). Any form of life consisting of different functional parts that are mutually interdependent.

orifice (or' i fis). An opening or mouth.

Orinase (or' in āz) Tolbutamide; an orally administered drug used in treatment of diabetes.

orthodontics (or thō don' tiks). Specialty that deals with diagnosing and treating irregularities of the developing teeth and occlusion, often by the placement of metal bands (braces) around the teeth.

osmosis (os mō' sis). The diffusion of fluids through membranes.

osseous (os' ē us). Bony.

osteitis (os tē ī' tis). Inflammation of bone.

osteoarthritis ((os tē ō ar thrī' tis). A degenerative form of arthritis that affects the articular surfaces of synovial joints.

osteogenic (os tē ō jen' ik). Bone producing.

osteolytic (os tē ō lit' ik). Bone destroying.

osteomalacia (os tē ō ma lā' shi a). Softening of the bony skeleton caused by deficiency of minerals and vitamin D.

osteomyelitis (os tē ō mī el ī' tis). A purulent inflammation of bone.

osteoporosis (os tē ō por ō' sis). Thinning of bone due to loss of calcium and phosphorus.

osteotome (os tē ō tōm). A chisel-like instrument for cutting bone.

osteotomy (os tē ŏt' ō mi). Surgical division of a bone.

otolaryngology (ō tō lar ing gol' ō ji). The branch of medicine that deals with the anatomy, function and diseases of the ear, nose and throat.

overbite (ō' ver bĭt). The vertical overlapping of the upper teeth to the lower.

ovulation (ov ū lā' shun). During a woman's menstrual cycle, it is the process of maturation and discharge of an ovum (egg).

oxidation (ok si dā' shun). The process whereby oxygen is added to a substance to produce oxides.

Oxycel (oks' i sel). Oxidized cellulose, used to promote clotting of a wound or incision.

oxygenation (oks i jen ā' shun). The enriching of a substance with oxygen.

pacemaker (pās ma' ker). An electrical device that is either implanted subcutaneously or worn externally, to regulate heart rate.

palate (pal' it). The roof of the mouth.

palliative (pal' i a tiv). Treatment of a disease that relieves symptoms, but does not cure it.

palpation (pal pā' shun). Manual examination.

palpitation (pal pi tā' shun). Forceful, rapid heart beat, which the patient is aware of.

panarthritis (pan ar thri' tis). Inflammation of the entire joint.

pandemic (pan dem' ik). The presence of a disease throughout an entire country or the world.

papillae (pa pil a). The short, hairlike projections of the tongue.

papilloma (pap i lō' ma). A benign tumor of nonglandular epithelial tissue.

papule (pap' ūl). A small pointed skin elevation.

paracentesis (par a sen tē' sis). The removal of fluid from a closed cavity, using a hollow needle.

paraformaldehyde (par a form al' di hīd). A powdery form of formaldehyde.

paralysis (par al' i sis). Partial or total loss of nervous function to part of the body. It may be motor or sensory or both, causing an inability to move or feel.

paranasal (par a nā' zal). Around or near the nasal cavities.

paraplegia (par a plē' ji a). Paralysis of the lower extremities and organs.

parasite (par' a sīt). An animal or plant that lives on or in another organism of a different species, and gets its nourishment from it's host.

Parasympathetic (par a sim pa thet' ik). That part of the autonomic nervous system that is derived from the cranial and sacral nerves that regulate involuntary body functions.

parenteral (par en' ter al). Taken into the body in a manner other than by mouth.

paresis (par ē' sis). Partial motor paralysis.

paresthesia (par es thēz' i a). Abnormal loss of sensation.

parotid gland (par o' tid gland). The salivary gland that is located in front of the ear.

parotitus (par o tī' tis). Inflammation of the parotid gland.

paroxysmal (par ok siz' mal). Recurring, sudden attacks.

partial (par' shal) or "partial denture." A denture that is used to replace some but not all missing teeth in either the upper or lower jaw.

patent (pat' ent). Open, not closed.

pathogen (path' ō gen). A living agent that causes disease.

pathognomonic (path og nō mon' ik). Characteristic of a particular disease.

pathology (pa thol ō ji). The science dealing with the causes and nature of diseases.

pedodontist (pē dō don' tist). A specialist in diagnosing and treating diseases of children's teeth.

pedunculated (pē dung kū lāt ed). Stalk-like.

pemphigus (pem' fig us). A disease that is characterized by bulla or blister formation on the skin and mucous membranes.

pentobarbital (pen tō bar' bit al). A short-acting barbiturate.

Pentothal (pen' tō thal). Thiopental; a short-acting barbituate, given by intravenous injection.

percussion (per kush' un). Tapping of an area to determine the fullness or resonance. In dentistry, one of the diagnostic tools to locate pain.

perforation (pur fō rā shun). A hole in a normally intact tissue.

periadenitis (per i a den ī' tis). Inflammation in the soft tissue around glands.

periapex (per i ā peks). The area surrounding the root tip of a tooth.

periarthritis (per i ar thrī tis). Inflammation of the tissue around a joint.

pericarditis (per i car dī' tis). Inflammation of the outer covering of the heart.

periodontal disease (per i ō don' tal di zēz). Disease of the gums.

periodontal pocket (per i ō don' tal pok' et). Seen in periodontal disease, this is a deep area between the tooth and the gingiva surrounding it.

periodontist (per i ō don' tist). A specialist in diagnosing and treating the periodontium (see below).

periodontitis (per i ō don tī' tis). An inflammatory and degenerative breakdown of the tissues around the teeth. Commonly known as "pyorrhea." Usually due to excessive calculus formation and malocclusion.

periodontium (per i ō don' shi um). The surrounding structures of the teeth, including gum, bone, ligament, and membrane.

periodontosis (per i ō don tō' sis). A severe periodontitis that is found in isolated, as opposed to generalized, locations; often in teenagers or juveniles.

periosteum (per i os' tē um). The membrane covering bones.

periostitis (per ī os tī' tis). Inflammation of the periosteum.

periostosis (per i os tō' sis). A bony growth that forms around existing bone.

peritrate (per' i trāt). Pentaerythritol tetranitrate; a coronary artery dilating medication.

perleche (per lesh'). A skin inflammation at the corners of the mouth.

pernicious anemia (per' nish ous a' nē mē a). Abnormally low red-blood cell count due to loss of protein produced by the gastric glands.

peroral (pur ō ral). Through the mouth.

pertussis (per tus' is). Whooping cough.

petechiae (pē tēk ē ī). Small hemorrhagic spots.

phagocyte (fag' ō sīt). A cell that engulfs debris and cells in the tissues.

pharmacology (far ma kol' ō ji). The science of drugs.

pharyngitis (far in jī' tis). Inflammation of the pharynx.

pharynx (far' inks). The opening that lies between the mouth and the esophagus.

phenacetin (fen as' et in). A valuable analgesic with low toxicity.

phenobarbital (fē nō bar' bit ol). A long-acting barbiturate.

phenol (fē nol). Carbolic acid; a strong antiseptic.

phenoxymethyl penicillin (fen oks i meth' il pen i sil' in). Penicillin V. Orally administered.

phenylbutazone (fen il bū' ta zōn). A strong analgesic and anti-inflammatory drug; toxic reactions are common.

phlegm (flem). Mucus originating in the bronchi.

phobia (fō bi a). Abnormal fear.

phosphorus (fos' fō rus). An important nonmetallic element found in nerve and bone tissue.

physiology (fiz ī ol' ō ji). The study of the functions of the body.

picrotoxin (pik rō toks' in). A central nervous system stimulant used to treat barbiturate poisoning.

pin amalgam (pin a mal' gam). A silver filling placed over metal pins embedded in a tooth to increase the retention of the filling.

273

pineal body (pin' ē al). A small structure located on the surface of the midbrain, whose function is still not understood.

pituitary gland (pi tū' i ter i gland). A small endocrine gland located in the skull. Its secretions regulate growth and metabolism.

placebo (pla sē' bo). An inert, chemically useless substance given as a substitute for medication.

plane of occlusion (plān ov o klŏŏ' zhun). An imaginary line representing the axis on which the teeth meet when biting.

plasma (plaz' ma). The fluid portion of blood.

platelets (plāt' letz). Also called thrombocytes. They are tiny solid particles in the blood and are important in clotting.

poliomyelitis (pōl i ō mī el ī' tis). Infantile paralysis caused by viral infection of the spinal cord and/or brain stem.

polyarteritis (pol i ar ter ī' tis). Inflammation of many arteries.

polycythemia (pol i sī thē' mi a). A marked increase in the number of circulating red blood cells.

polymorphonuclear (pol i mor fō nū' klē ar). Characterized by a multilobulated nucleus; usually refers to the granulocytes that are 70 percent of the total white blood cells.

polyp (pol' ip). A stalk-like, usually benign, tumor of mucous membranes.

pontic (pon' tik). Term used to describe the replacement for lost teeth in a bridge. Abutments are used for support on both sides of the pontic.

porcelain (pōr' se lin). Material used to fabricate false teeth or baked over a cast crown that is fabricated from Kaolin, feldspar, quartz and other minerals to match the color of the remaining teeth.

porcelain jacket crown (por' se lin jak' it kroun). A crown used on anterior teeth; not a "cap." (See Ill. page 275.)

post (post). A cast or ready-made prosthesis that fills the finished root canal, which is then built up with a core for later coverage by a crown.

prefrontal (prē frun tal). Located in the anterior section of the frontal lobe of the cerebrum.

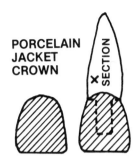

PORCELAIN
JACKET
CROWN

X SECTION

premedication (prē med ik ā' shun). A drug that is administered before another drug to enhance or modify its action.

premolar (prē mō' lar). Teeth between the canines and the molars; used for grinding. They have two cusps (and are sometimes called bicuspids). They have either one or two roots.

pressor (pres' er). A drug that raises blood pressure.

primary teeth (prī mer i tēth). See *deciduous teeth.*

prognathism (prog' na thiz m). Condition where the lower jaw is abnormally forward in relation to the upper.

prognosis (prog nō' sis). A prediction of the probable course and outcome of a disease.

prolapse (prō' laps). The dropping or falling of a structure.

pronate (prō' nāt). To turn the ventral surface of a body structure downward to assume a prone position.

prophylaxis (prō fi lak sis). A thorough cleaning of the teeth; commonly abbreviated to "prophy." This includes scaling to remove the calculus that has formed.

prosthesis (pros' thē sis). An artificial replacement for a part of the body. In dentistry, this usually refers to bridges, crowns or dentures.

protease (prō' tē az). Any protein-digesting enzyme.

prothrombin (prō throm' bin). The substance formed in the liver, which is the precursor of thrombin; it occurs in blood plasma. *Prothrombin time* is the measure of its concentration in the blood.

proximal (prok' si mal). Term used to describe any tooth surface that touches another tooth.

pruritus (prōō ri' tus). Itching.

psychogenic (sī kō jen' ik). Caused by the mind.

psychosis (sī kō' sis). Mental illness that involves a loss of contact with reality.

ptyalin (tī a lin). The salivary gland enzyme that converts starch into dextrin and maltose.

ptyalolith (tī' a lō lith). Salivary calculus or stone.

pulmonary (pul' mō ner i). Relating to the lungs.

pulp (pulp). The innermost layer of the tooth consisting of connective tissue, blood vessels and nerves. The blood vessels nourish the tooth, whereas the nerves transmit sensation of pain to the brain.
The pulp has two chambers, the pulp chamber and the root canal. The pulp chamber lies in the top (crown) of the tooth. The root canal is in the root. Blood vessels and nerves enter the root canal through a small opening at the tip of the root, extend through the root canal and into the pulp chamber.

pulp cap (pulp kap). A protective lining inserted when caries removal necessitates injury to the pulp. It is placed next to the pulp with the anticipation of healing and forming new dentin.

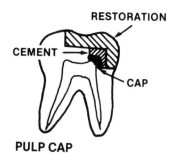

PULP CAP

pulse (puls). The impulse transmitted to arteries by the contraction of the left ventricle of the heart. It is used to measure the frequency and regularity of the heart beat.

puncture (pungk tur). A stab or incision made with a sharp, pointed instrument to inject or withdraw fluid.

purpura (pur' pū ra). The leakage of blood from capillaries into the skin or mucous membranes. It is characterized by small or large red spots under the skin.

purulent (pū rŏŏ lent). Relating to pus.

pus (pus). A yellowish liquid containing bacteria and white blood cells. It develops from infections.

pyemia (pī ē' mi a). A serious condition in which living bacteria are pathologically present in the blood stream and then lodge and grow in different organs, forming abscesses.

pyogenic (pī ō jen' ik). Referring to pus formation.

pyorrhea (pī' o rē a). Inflammation of the tooth sockets and surrounding gum tissue, resulting in a loosening of the teeth.

pyrexia (pī rēk' si a). Fever.

quadrant (kwod' rant). One of four divisions of the mouth—either upper right, upper left, lower right, or lower left.

UPPER RIGHT QUADRANT

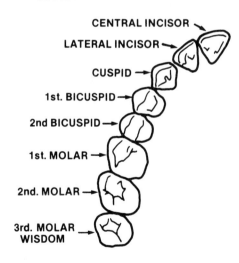

CENTRAL INCISOR
LATERAL INCISOR
CUSPID
1st. BICUSPID
2nd BICUSPID
1st. MOLAR
2nd. MOLAR
3rd. MOLAR WISDOM

quadrant dentistry (kwod' rant den' tis tri). The treatment of dental disease by each section of the mouth, to minimize the number of visits.

quadriplegia (kwod ri plē' ji a). The condition in which both arms and both legs are paralyzed.

quinidine (kwin' i dīn). Chemical used to treat atrial fibrillation of the heart. It is similar to quinine.

quinsy (kwin' zi). Sore throat. A condition characterized by acute inflammation of the tonsil, and abscess formation next to it.

radioactive (rā di ō ak' tiv). Any material that emits rays (such as radium, radioactive forms of gold, iodine and mercury). It is used for investigation, when certain illnesses are suspected.

radiography (rā di og' ra fi). The taking of X-rays (radiographs).

radiologist (rā di ol' ō jist). A physician who specializes in using X-rays to diagnose and treat illnesses.

radiopaque (ra di ō pak'). Material that cannot be penetrated by X-rays. Enamel is radiopaque.

radiotherapy (rā di ō ther' a pē). Treatment by X-ray or radioactive material.

ranula (ran' ū la). A swelling caused by a cyst of one of the salivary glands underneath the tongue.

reagent (rē ā' jent). A substance used to produce a chemical reaction.

receptor (rē sep' tor). Part of a nerve ending that receives and transmits stimuli.

recumbent (rē kum' bent). Lying down.

reflex (rē' fleks). A response to a stimulus that is involuntary. Such responses as blinking, sneezing, or coughing are reflexes.
The *Babinski reflex* is tested when the sole of the foot is scratched. It often indicates disease of the brain or spinal cord.

refraction (rē frak' shun). The testing of the eyes by an opthalmologist or optometrist for the prescribing of glasses.

refractory (rē frak' tō ri). An illness that does not respond to treatment.

regurgitation (rē gur ji tā' shun). A backward flow, as from the stomach to the mouth.

remission (rē mish' un). A period during an illness when the symptoms disappear.

renal (rē' nal). Pertaining to the kidneys.

resection (rē sek' shun). Removal or excision by surgery.

reserpine (rē ser' pin). Also called a rauwolfia alkaloid; used to treat high blood pressure, and as a tranquilizer.

residual (rē zid' ū al). Material left behind, such as air left in the lung after forced expiration.

resistance (rē zis' tins). Power to withstand or resist; the body's ability to fight off infection.

resonance (rez' ō nans). When the chest is percussed, the vibrations heard when the lungs are clear and filled with air.

respiration (res pi rā' shun). The act of breathing.

respirator (res' pi rā tor). A machine that artificially causes the lungs to inflate and deflate; an "iron lung."

respiratory failure (re spir' a tō ri fāl ūr). A condition in which the lungs fail to oxygenate the blood.

resuscitation (rē sus' i tā shun). The process of reviving a person who is near death, or dead. *Mouth-to-mouth resuscitation* involves the rescuer breathing into the victim's mouth.

retention (rē ten' shun). The condition of holding in—as in the retention of urine. It is a description, in dentistry, of the property and techniques of a filling, to insure the material remains in place.

reticular (rĕ tik' ū lar). A structure that resembles a net.

reticulocyte (re tik' ū lō sīt). A red blood cell that is immature and still contains some of the nucleus that was present in its early stages of development.

reticuloendothelial system (ret ik' ū lō end oth ē li al sis' tem). All of the white blood cells that ingest bacteria and other foreign bodies. They are found in the bone marrow, liver and lymph nodes of the body.

retina (ret' i na). The innermost layers of the eyeball upon which light rays are focused.

retractor (rē trak' tor). A type of instrument, of which there are many, that is used to pull back the tissue so that the surgeon is able to see underlying areas. Retraction of soft tissue in the oral cavity is often accomplished with a mouth mirror, cotton rolls or mechanical devices.

retrograde (ret' rō grād). To flow backward, or in the opposite direction from normal. In dentistry, a retrograde filling involves the apex of the tooth.

retrogression (ret rō gresh' un). Regression; a degeneration or deterioration of tissue.

retroverted (ret rō vĕr' ted). Tilted or turned backward.

RH factor (R H fak' ter). This is a substance or component of the blood. People whose blood contains this substance are "Rh-positive." Those who do not (15 percent of the population) are "Rh-negative." Presence or absence is an inherited characteristic.
Problems arise when an Rh-negative mother is pregnant with an Rh-positive fetus. This condition may lead to her losing the child. All pregnant mothers should be tested for the Rh factor.

rheumatic fever (rū' mat ik fe' ver). A disease, usually of children, that is inflammatory in nature; patient often runs a high fever, has swelling of the joints that can be quite painful and has inflamed heart muscles and valves. Initial infection is a strep (streptococcus) infection of the throat.

rheumatic heart disease (rū' mat ik hārt di zez'). Heart disease resulting from a rheumatic fever infection of the valves and muscles of the heart. The mitral valve and the aortic valve are usually affected. Dental patients who have had RHD are commonly put on antibiotic premedication.

rheumatism (roo' ma tiz m). A term used to cover a group of diseases affecting the joints, tendons, bones or muscles.

rheumatoid arthritis (roo' ma toid ar thri' tis). Disease in which joints are affected. Ill health and crippling joint deformities occur.

rhinitis (ri nī' tis). The condition in which the lining of the nose, the mucous membranes, become inflamed. May be caused by an allergic reaction.

rhinoplasty (rī' nō plas ti). Plastic surgery of the nose.

riboflavin (rī bō flā' ven). Vitamin B_2. Lack of B_2 causes skin cracking and inflammation of the eyes and tongue.

ribonucleic acid (RNA) (rī' bō nu klē ik as' id). This substance, plus deoxyribonucleic acid (DNA) is found in every living cell. It is the portion of the nucleus of the cell that reproduces itself, thereby transmitting all inherited characteristics.

rickets (ri' kets). Disease of infants generally associated with a deficiency of Vitamin D. May cause bowed legs or malformation of the chest.

Ritalin (ri ta lin). Methyphenidate; an antidepressant.

Rocky Mountain spotted fever (rok' ē moun' ten spot' ed fē' ver). A disease caused by rickettsia, in the typhus group. These parasites are carried by ticks.

Roentgen rays (ront' gen rā z). X-rays, named for Wilhem von Roentgen, a German physicist who died in 1923.

root (root). The part of the tooth found below the gum line, containing blood vessels and nerves.

root canal therapy. (root ka nal' ther' a pē). This involves the removal of the pulp of a tooth, because it has become infected. After the pulp has been removed, the dentist fills the canal.

Rorschack test (ror' shak test). A psychological test in which a specific set of ink blots is interpreted by a patient, and a diagnosis is made based on these interpretations. Named for a Swiss psychiatrist who died in 1922.

roseola (rō zē ō' la). German measles; rose-colored spots appear on the skin and a fever.

roughage (ruf' aj). The indigestible fibers such as cellulose that are not absorbed from the intestine. Provides bulk in the diet, which helps to stimulate peristalsis and elimination.

rubefacient (roo bi fa' shent). A substance that reddens the skin when applied to it.

rubber dam (rub er dam). A perforated rubber sheet clamped to the teeth for isolation during dental procedures.

rubella (roo bel' a). German measles. A contagious viral infection characterized by fever, rash, upper-respiratory symptoms and swollen glands.

rubeola (rū bē ō' la). Measles. A highly infectious disease spread by droplet infection. Characterized by high fever and rash beginning on the face and upper neck. Differs from rubella by a longer duration of the rash, and a higher fever.

rugae (roo' jē) Fold-like wrinkles.

sac (sak). A small cavity or pouch.

saccharin (sak' a rin). A chemical substitute for sugar, containing fewer calories.

sagittal (saj' it al). The front-to-back plane of the body.

salicylic acid (sal i sil' ik as' id). A fungicidal and bacteriostatic chemical. Aspirin.

saline (sā' līn). A salt-and-water solution. Normal saline is 0.9 percent salt.

saliva (sal ī' va). The sticky secretion of the salivary glands.

sanguineous (sang gwin' i us). Bloody; blood red.

sarcoidosis (sar koid ō' sis). A disease of unknown cause, characterized by tubercular-like lesions of the skin, lymph glands and other organs.

sarcoma (sar kō' ma). Malignant growth of connective tissue, muscle or bone.

scaler (skāl' er). Instrument used to remove hard deposits from the teeth in periodontal therapy.

scapula (skap' ū la). The shoulder blade.

Scarlet fever (skar' let fē' ver). An infection caused by streptococci, usually in children. Characterized by sore throat, fever and rash.

sciatica (sī at' i ka). Pain along the distribution of the sciatic nerve, the buttock, the thigh, the calf and the foot.

scirrhus (skir' us). A hard carcinoma.

sclera (sklē ra). The white of the eye.

scleroderma (skler o dur' ma). A skin disease causing hard patches with color changes. It may affect other body organs.

sclerosis (sklē rō sis). Abnormal hardening of a tissue.

scoliosis (skō li ō' sis). Abnormal spinal curvature.

scorbutic (skor bū' tik). Referring to scurvy, caused by severe vitamin C shortage.

seborrhea (seb o rē' a). A skin condition caused by overactivity of the sebaceous glands.

secretion (sē krē' shun). A substance formed or found in a gland, and that is passed into the blood stream, the gastrointestinal tract or to the outside of the body.

sedative (sed' a tiv). A substance that decreases activity of the body.

semicomatose (sem i kō' ma tōs). Almost unconscious.

senescence (sē nes' ens). The normal mental and physical changes of aging.

senile (sē nīl). Aging accompanied by degenerative changes, mentally and physically.

sepsis (sep' sis). The condition of infection by purulent organisms.

septum (sep' tum). The partition between cavities, including the bone that separates the teeth.

sequestrum (sē kwes' trum). A piece of necrotic bone, separated from normal bone but still retained in the tissue.

serum (sēr um). The liquid residue when blood clots.

sessile (ses' il). With a broad base.

shock (shok). Severe injury or illness may cause this reduction in blood volume, leading to rapid pulse, blood pressure drop, pallor and clammy skin.

shunt (shunt). The passage of blood through nonnormal channels.

sialagogue (sī al' a gog). A substance that increases salivary flow.

sialolith (sī a' lō lith). A stone in a salivary gland or duct.

Sickle-cell anemia (sik' l sel a nē mē a). A hereditary anemia, found chiefly in Blacks, and characterized by crescent-shaped red cells.

sign (sīn). Any observable evidence of disease.

sinus (sī' nus). A hollow or cavity.

slough (sluf). Necrotic tissue that becomes separated from healthy tissue.

smear (smēr). A thin film of material spread out on a glass slide for microscopic examination.

sodium chloride (sō' di um klōr' ĭd). Salt, normally present in body tissue.

solute (sol' ūt). Material found dissolved in a liquid.

solvent (sol' vent). Any material in which a substance is dissolved.

soporific (so pō rif ik). A substance that produces a deep sleep.

space maintainer (spās mān tān' r). An appliance that maintains space between deciduous teeth when early loss occurs. Allows space for proper eruption of permanent teeth.

SPACE MAINTAINER

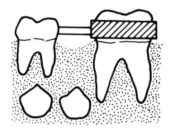

spansule (span shūl). A chemical preparation that releases controlled amounts of drugs over a period of time when administered orally.

spasm (spaz' m). Involuntary, convulsive muscle contractions.

spatula (spat' ū la). A flat, flexible knife-like instrument used to spread and mix chemical substances.

spectrophotometer (spek trō fō tom' e ter). An instrument used to measure the relative intensity of varying parts of a light spectrum.

sphenoid (sfē' noid). The wedge-shaped bone located at the base of the skull.

sphincter (sfingk' ter). A circular muscle, which upon contraction, closes an orifice or opening.

spirochete (spī' rō kēt). A spiral-shaped bacterium.

spleen (splēn). A lymphoid organ located at the tail of the pancreas, behind the stomach, which aids in the recycling of red blood cells.

spore (spor). A stage in the life cycle of certain bacteria in which the cell becomes encapsulated, and life almost stops.

sputum (spū' tum). Saliva mixed with material expectorated from the lungs.

squamous (skwa' mous). Scaly. Refers to the epithelial covering of the skin.

stapes (stā' pēz). A stirrup-shaped bone of the middle ear.

staphylococcus (staf i lō kok' us). A genus of bacteria, which includes a number of toxin-producing types.

stasis (stā' sis). Stopping of movement or motion.

stenosis (ste nō' sis). A narrowing.

sterile (ster' il). Free from microorganisms.

sternum (stur' num). The breast bone.

steroids (ster' oids). A naturally occurring group of chemicals that include sex hormones, adrenocortical hormones and bile acids. The term now includes synthetic analogues of the adrenocortical hormones.

stomatitis (stō ma tī' tis). Inflammation of the mucous membrane lining the oral cavity.

stone (stōn) A hardened mineral mass.

strangulation (strang gū lā' shun). Constriction of a structure leading to a circulatory impediment.

streptococcus (strep tō kok' us). A genus of toxin-producing bacteria that causes many infections in man.

streptomycin (strep tō mi' sin). An antibiotic primarily used to treat tuberculosis.

stricture (strick' tūr). A narrowing of a canal or tube.

stroke (strōk). Term used to identify the result of a cerebrovascular accident. It usually includes hemiplegia, or the paralysis of one side of the body.

stupor (stū' por). Marked impairment, just short of unconsciousness.

subacute (sub ak ūt'). Moderately severe.

subcutaneous (sub kū tā' ni us). Under the skin.

subliminal (sub lim' in al). Just below the level of perception.

sublingual (sub lin' gwal). Under the tongue.

subluxation (sub luks ā' shun). Incomplete dislocation of a joint.

submucosa (sub mū kō' sa). The connective tissue layer just below the mucous membrane.

subperiosteal (sub per i os' ti al). Beneath the membrane that covers bone.

sulfonamides (sul fon' a midz). A group of orally administered bacteriostatic agents.

super eruption (soo' per e rup' shun). A condition that occurs when a tooth is lost, and the opposing tooth overerupts (or extrudes).

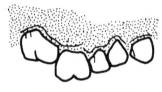

SUPER ERUPTION

super numerary. (soo' per nū' mer er i). An extra tooth.

supinate (sū' pi nāt). To lie face up, or turn palm up.

suppuration (sup ū rā' shun). Pus formation.

surface of the teeth (sur' fis of the' tēth). Reference point on any given tooth—refers to points toward the midline of mouth (mesial), away from midline of mouth (distal), biting edge (incisal), masticating surface (occlusal), cheek surface (buccal), tongue surface (lingual), and lip surface (labial). (See Ill. page 287.)

suture (sū' tŭr). A stitch; also, the junction of the cranial bones.

sympathetic (sim pa thet' ik). The part of the autonomic nervous system that ennervates plain muscle.

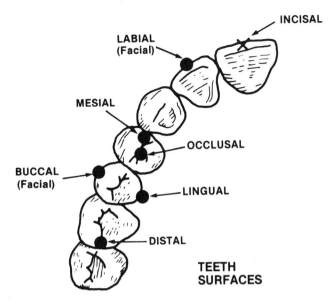

TEETH
SURFACES

symphysis (sim' fi sis). The growing together or fibro-carti-laginous union of two bones.

syncope (sing' ko pi). Fainting.

syndrome (sin' drōm). A group of signs or symptoms that, col-lectively, are typical of a specific disease.

synovial membrane (sī nō' vi al mem' brān). The membrane that lines the joints.

tachycardia (tak i kar' di a). Unusually rapid heartbeat.

tactile (tak' tīl). Relating to the sense of touch.

tantalum (tant a lum). A tissue-compatible metal, used to help repair defects in the body, including dental implants and prostheses.

tartar (tar' tar). Same as *calculus*.

tegument (teg' ū ment). The outer covering; in the case of hu-man beings it is the skin of the body.

telangiectasis (tel an ji ek' ta sis). Dilation of the surface capil-laries on the body.

tendon (ten' don). The tough, white cord that attaches muscle to bone.

thiamine (thī' a min). Vitamin B_1.

thiopental (thī ō pen' tal). A barbiturate, injected intravenously to initiate anesthesia.

thoracic (tho' ras' ik). Relating to the chest cavity.

thorax (thor' aks). The chest cavity.

Thorazine (thor' a zēn). Chlorpromazine; one of the major tranquilizers, used in the treatment of psychosis.

thrombin (throm' bin). The product derived from prothrombin in the blood-clotting process that aids in the healing process.

three-quarter crown (thrē kwor'ter kroun). Cast-gold restoration covering approximately three quarters of the tooth.

**3/4 CAST GOLD
CROWN**

thrombocytopenia (throm bō sī tō pē' nē a). Reduced number of blood platelets.

thromboembolism (throm bō em' bō lism). The blockage of a blood vessel by a clot carried there from a blood vessel in another part of the body.

thrombosis (throm bō' sis). The process or formation of a blood clot within a blood vessel.

thrombus (throm' bus). The blood clot formed within a blood vessel.

thrush (thrush). A candidia or fungus infection found in the mouth, usually in infants.

thymus (thī mus) A small gland located behind the breast bone. It is ductless.

thyroid (thī'royd). The endocrine gland located on both sides of the trachea. It controls metabolic rate.

thyroxine (thī roks' in). The chief hormone produced by the thyroid gland.

tic-douloreux (tik dōō ler oo'). Trigeminal neuralgia—severely painful spasms which can occur along the trigeminal nerve in any of its three divisions. Usually, they touch a so-called "trigger zone" resulting in excruciating pain.

tolerance (tol' er ans). The ability to withstand the action of a drug.

toxemia (toks e' mī a). Generalized tissue poisoning caused by bacterial infection or trauma.

toxin (tok' sin). A poisonous product of bacterial infection that, when injected into the body, causes the formation of an antibody or antitoxin.

toxoid (tok' soid). A toxin that has been modified so that its poisonous effects are eliminated, but its antigenic-producing properties are retained.

trachea (tra' kē a). The windpipe.

tracheotomy (trā kē ot' ō mē). An incision in the anterior wall of the trachea to allow for insertion of a device to restore breathing capability.

trans- (trans). The prefix meaning "through."

trauma (tro' ma). Physical or emotional injury.

tremor (trem' or). Involuntary trembling.

trephine (tre fĭn'). A surgical instrument used to remove a circular piece of bone or soft tissue. Trephination is a boring of hole(s) through the skull.

Treponema (trep o nē' ma). A spiral-shaped bacterium. Among the diseases caused by members of this species are syphilis and yaws.

triamcinolone (try am sin' ō lōne). An anti-inflammatory steroid.

trismus (triz' mus). A spasm of the mastriatory muscles causing inability to open the mouth.

trophic (trof' ik). Relating to nutrition.

trypsin (trip' sin}. A pancreatic enzyme.

tuberculosis (tū ber kū lō' sis). A highly infectious disease caused by mycobacterium tuberculosis.

tumescence (tu mes' ens). A condition of swelling.

tumor (tū' mor). An abnormal mass of tissue that does not exhibit a useful function.

tussis (tus' is). A cough.

tympanum (tim' pan um). The middle-ear cavity.

ulcer (ul' ser). An open sore in a body surface.

ultrasonic (ul' tra son' ik). High-frequency sound waves that are inaudible to the human ear. Also, in dentistry, a method of removing debris from instruments, and scaling calculus from teeth using these sound waves.

urticaria (ur ti kā' ri a). An allergic skin reaction that disappears after a brief period of time, leaving no visible trace.

uvula (ū vū la). The center, posterior tab that hangs from the soft palate.

varicose vein (va' ri kōs vān). A dilated vein with incompetent valves, leading to impaired blood flow.

variola (va rī ō la). Smallpox.

vascular (vas' cū lar). Supplied with blood vessels.

vector (vek' tor). Disease carrier.

venipuncture (vē ni pungk tūr). Insertion of a needle into a vein.

venous (vē' nus). Referring to the veins.

venule (ven' ūl). A small vein.

verruca (ve rōō' ka). Wart.

vertigo (ver' ti gō). Dizziness.

vesicle (ves' ik l). A small, hollow structure.

vesiculitis (ves ik ū lī' tis). Inflammation of a vesicle.

vestigial (ves ti' gī al). Rudimentary.

viricidal (vī ri sī' dal). Capable of killing a virus.

virus (vī' rus). A submicroscopic organism that exists within living cells, and causes disease.

viscera (vis' er a). The internal organs.

vitreous (vit' re us). Jellylike.

weal (wēl). Surface blister.

xeroderma (zē rō der' ma). Dry skin.

xerostomia (zē ros tō' mi a). Dry mouth.

X-rays (x rāz). There are various methods used to X-ray a patient's mouth. One is the full-mouth survey, which requires 14 exposures of all quadrants of the mouth, showing one to three entire teeth on each exposure. This allows the dentist to see beneath the surface.
The second type is the "bite wing" X-ray survey, with a series of from two to four exposures of crowns of posterior teeth showing interproximal areas. This is used to check for dental caries.

xylocaine (zī' lō kān). Lidocaine; a local anesthetic.